CREATING UNIQUE COPIES

Human Reproductive Cloning, Uniqueness, and Dignity

Evangelos D. Protopapadakis

CREATING UNIQUE COPIES
HUMAN REPRODUCTIVE CLONING, UNIQUENESS, AND DIGNITY

with a foreword by
Roberto Andorno

Logos Verlag Berlin

Evangelos D. Protopapadakis

Creating Unique Copies:
Human Reproductive Cloning, Uniqueness, and Dignity

Bibliographic information published by
the Deutsche Nationalbibliothek.
The Deutsche Nationalbibliothek lists this publication
in the Deutsche Nationalbibliografie;
detailed bibliographic data are available in the Internet at
http://dnb.d-nb.de.

ISBN 978-3-8325-5698-3
Logos Verlag Berlin GmbH
Georg-Knorr-Str. 4, Geb. 10
D-12681 Berlin
Germany

Tel.: +49 (0)30 42 85 10 90
Fax: +49 (0)30 42 85 10 92
www.logos-verlag.com

To my brother.

TABLE OF CONTENTS

Foreword

In 1997, Ian Wilmut and colleagues from the Roslin Institute in Scotland published an article in *Nature* announcing the birth of Dolly the sheep, the first mammal to be cloned from an adult somatic cell.[1] The paper immediately made headlines around the world and raised serious concerns among ethicists and policymakers about the nightmarish prospect that the same procedure could be soon used to create genetically (and physically) identical human beings. In response to those concerns, intergovernmental organizations such as the United Nations, UNESCO, and the Council of Europe adopted policies to prevent that prospect from becoming a reality. Simultaneously, several countries did the same at the domestic level. But ethicists and legal scholars still had to face difficult theoretical questions: Do we have a right to the uniqueness of our genetic information? Are we entitled to predetermine the genetic makeup of our children? What value should we attach to sexual reproduction, that is, to the natural process by which every human being is conceived through the unique combination of genetic material from two different individuals? Does the present generation have a duty to preserve the integrity and identity of humankind?[2]

---

[1] Ian Wilmut, et al., "Viable Offspring Derived from Fetal and Adult Mammalian Cells," *Nature* 385, no. 6619 (1997): 810-813.

[2] In the early 2000s, I had the opportunity to discuss some of those questions. See "Réflexions sur le clonage humain dans une perspective éthico-juridique et de droit comparé," *Les Cahiers de droit* 43, no. 1 (2001): 129:145, https://www.erudit.org/fr/revues/cd1/2001-v42-n1-cd3825/043632ar.pdf; "Biomedicine and International Human Rights Law: In Search of a Global Consensus," *Bulletin of the World Health Organization* 80, no. 12 (2002): 959-963, https://apps.who.int/iris/handle/10665/268678.

This book brings attention back to those difficult questions relating to cloning that have been to some extent forgotten in recent literature. While this foreword will not delve into all the nuanced arguments presented in the book, it will briefly touch on two main objections to human reproductive cloning: uniqueness and dignity. Through examination of both arguments, Protopapadakis ultimately concludes that they "do not suffice to convince us that cloning should not be considered a morally legitimate reproductive option."

I do not share this skeptical conclusion. The uniqueness of every human individual is closely linked to the very notion of "person." Throughout history, being a "person" has meant being a unique entity (a human individual) that has inherent value and cannot be reduced to a mere object. As Kant put it, a "person" cannot be replaced by something else as its equivalent precisely because he or she possesses "dignity" and not a "price."[3] It is true that the cloned individual would be a truly distinct person from his or her "model" (the cell donor) and from other "copies" that could have been produced from that same DNA. In other words, each clone would possess his or her own dignity, just like any other human being. However, the circumstance of being physically identical to other people would very likely pose a significant risk for his or her psychological identity; it will also be at odds with the legitimate interest of other individuals and society at large in being able to distinguish who is who. Our physical appearance, particularly our face, is not a minor or insignificant element of our personality. In fact, it strengthens our self-awareness and sense of self, as our body is the most direct and visible manifestation of our uniqueness.

---

[3] Immanuel Kant, *Grundlegung zur Metaphysik der Sitten,* in *Kant Werke,* vol. IV (Wiesbaden: Insel Verlag, 1956), 68.

There is almost no need to mention that the natural occurrence of monozygotic twins does not provide per se a justification for reproductive cloning. Not only because there is a fundamental difference between a *fact of nature*, for which nobody is responsible if it results in any harm, and a *human action*, which always is a source of responsibility, but because the mere fact that a certain phenomenon happens in nature does not necessarily authorize us to cause it *intentionally.* An earthquake that causes thousands of deaths is a perfectly natural phenomenon, and no one would deduce from it that we have the right to trigger the same dramatic result in order, for instance, to test the efficacy of a new weapon of mass destruction...[4]

Regarding human dignity, it is worth noting that this notion is often cited as the primary objection to reproductive cloning. This position is reflected in numerous international and domestic documents that prohibit this practice. It seems that we all share an underlying sense that creating genetically identical individuals is fundamentally problematic. Although it may be difficult to articulate precisely why, we intuitively recognize that reproductive cloning undermines a key aspect of human identity: our uniqueness and the inherent value of each of us.

Looking back on history, we may observe that the concept of dignity was traditionally used in bioethical discussions to highlight the intrinsic value of every individual (for instance, of participants in medical research). However, in the late 1990s,

---

[4] Additionally, monozygotic twins are an extremely rare occurrence, with only about 3 in 1,000 births. However, in reproductive cloning, there is no limit to the number of genetic "copies" that can be made of an individual, potentially resulting in dozens, hundreds, or thousands of clones. This would exponentially increase the risk of individuals having a diluted sense of identity.

human dignity began to be utilized to articulate disquiet about biotechnological developments, such as reproductive cloning and germline alteration, that may negatively impact *humanity as a whole.* In this more recent context, what is at stake is not so much the dignity of existing *individuals*, but the value we attach to the identity and integrity of the human species as such, that is, the *dignity of humankind.* It is important to mention that a purely human rights approach is powerless to face these new challenges because human rights are, by definition, only enjoyed by *existing* individuals, not by future people. This is why the well-intentioned claims often made that people have a "right not to be conceived as a genetic copy of another person" or a "right to inherit non-manipulated genetic information" are conceptually flawed.

The point I want to make is that the instruments dealing with bioethics that have been adopted since the end of the 1990s directly appeal to *human dignity*, and not to human rights, to ban human reproductive cloning and germline gene editing.[5] Three examples illustrate this trend: the UNESCO Universal Declaration on the Human Genome and Human Rights of 1997, which emphasizes the need to preserve the human genome as a "heritage of humanity" (Article 1), and expressly labels human reproductive cloning as "contrary to human dignity" (Article 11); the UN Declaration on Human Cloning of 2005, which calls on Member States "to prohibit all forms of human cloning inasmuch as they are incompatible with human dignity and the protection of human life" (Paragraph d); and the 1998 Additional Protocol to the Council of Europe Convention on Biomedicine and Human

---

[5] Roberto Andorno, "Human Dignity and Human Rights," in *Handbook of Global Bioethics,* eds. Henk ten Have, and Bert Gordijn, 45-57 (Dordrecht: Springer, 2014).

Rights, which prohibits human reproductive cloning on the grounds that it is "contrary to human dignity" (Preamble).

In conclusion, although I do not agree with all of Protopapadakis' arguments, I find his book to be a stimulating and thought-provoking read. It rekindles a vital discussion that has been largely overlooked by bioethicists over the past two decades or so. What is more, by thoroughly examining the objections raised against human reproductive cloning, the volume demonstrates that the underlying philosophical concerns are far more intricate than they initially appear.

Roberto Andorno
University of Zurich, Switzerland

Preface

My involvement with human reproductive cloning dates back to 2010, when I set out to write a book on the subject and its potential impact on a range of rights. The book was published in Greek in 2013, and I must admit that my current book has benefited greatly from my original research. The publication of the book was followed by a series of articles on the possible impact that the moral acceptance of cloning and its subsequent legalization might have on some of the rights of human beings, until I felt that everything I had to contribute to the debate on the interaction of cloning and rights had already been said. Still, I could not shake the thought that by limiting my research to rights, I was overlooking the forest and focusing instead on the tree: Rights do not arise spontaneously, nor do they flourish in a vacuum; rather, they require a solid rationale and a supporting network of concepts. That is, to the question "Why do people (or future generations or chipmunks or whatever) have this or that right?" it is not enough to answer, "Because they do," or "Because they are people (or future generations or chipmunks or whatever)." That would beg the question, and it is too simplistic a fallacy to fall for.

It also means that the debate over human reproductive cloning needs to go much deeper beneath the surface, where rights reside, and examine whether such technological advances, if accepted and legitimized, would call into question something much larger: Namely, the key concepts on which rights are based. If be it so, one could argue that while human reproductive cloning does not pose the slightest threat to this or that specific right – that is more or less the conclusion I have so far reached in my inquiry – it might nonetheless be morally reprehensible because it poses a threat to, or undermines, the concepts that underpin the rights under discussion.

In my view, the key concept that grounds and justifies all rights is *dignity*, a quality that human beings – for some, even *only* human beings – are supposed to possess. As Immanuel Kant famously argued, every rational nature possesses this quality because, by virtue of reason, it is capable of escaping the shackles and limitations of natural heteronomy and becoming a "universally legislative member for a merely possible realm of ends," i.e., a "will giving universal law," and thus "a law to itself (independently of all properties of the objects of volition)." Kant calls this capacity, which only rational beings possess, *autonomy*, and thinks of it as "the ground of the dignity of man and of every rational nature." Dignity in this sense is what makes every human being unique, in a way that non-human animals and things cannot be: Every rational nature is unique in that it becomes a law unto itself; by virtue of this, dignity – and thus, uniqueness – forms the perfect line of demarcation: Humans – along with every other rational nature – are accorded inherent value, while non-rational creatures can only have a *price*. The human being alone is "exalted above all price," and in this sense the human being is irreplaceable and indispensable, in a word, *unique*. This could also be true the other way around: If a certain creature is indispensable, irreplaceable, and unique, then it is "exalted above all price," and therefore the quality of dignity can be accorded to it; and conversely, if it is not indispensable, irreplaceable, and unique, the quality of dignity cannot be accorded to it. In view of the above, uniqueness and dignity seem to be inextricably intertwined, or rather mutually dependent.

Given the unprecedented importance that the Kantian concepts of dignity and autonomy have acquired, especially in the aftermath of the Holocaust, it is not surprising that – at least if we were to rely on the wording of universal declarations on human reproductive cloning, human dignity is considered in some way, and to a considerable extent, also as dependent on uniqueness. Uniqueness and dignity are concepts familiar particularly to Kantian ethicists, but not only to them; both are also key elements of other influential moral traditions. In the case of early utilitarians, for instance, and especially in John Stuart Mill's outlook, dignity takes the form of individuality, upon which the liberty of humans is based. At the same time, the Christian tradition that permeates the ethics of the Western world also holds to the doctrine that every human being is unique, a "hypostasis distinct by reason of [his or her] dignity," as Thomas has put it. Whether implicit or explicit, the assumed connection between uniqueness, dignity and the human condition has become the backbone of Western ethics.

Then, given that – by definition – human reproductive cloning aims to produce duplicates, that is human beings who are phenotypically and genetically identical to an existing – or once existed – human being, it may actually seem to threaten human dignity indeed, because it calls into question the uniqueness of human individuals. This is exactly what the book you are holding in your hands seeks to explore. Again, the focus largely seems to be on particular rights, but this is only because rights, as will be explained in subsequent chapters, are generally based on the concept of human dignity.

My expectations for this book cannot be different from those of any ethicist who decides to actively participate in any ethical debate: My wish for the journey on which I am about to embark is that it will contribute, at least to some extent, to the debate on human reproductive cloning and its implications for our uniqueness, dignity and rights; that it will bring the debate closer to a successful conclusion, whatever that may be. But even if it fails in doing so – the odds are always against such undertakings – may the journey at least stimulate and provoke reflection.

Evangelos D. Protopapadakis

1. Seeking Wisdom in the Definition of the Terms

The phrase "the beginning of wisdom is the definition of terms" is usually attributed to Socrates, but it seems that it was probably the Cynic philosopher Antisthenes who first introduced an aphorism very similar to this one.[1] The question of the origins of the aphorism, however, is likely to be of interest only to scholars: The view that before any debate the terms should be defined in advance as fully as possible, "as in the measuring of corn we place first the examination of the measure,"[2] as Epictetus puts it, runs through all classical and Hellenistic philosophical thought, as is evident in Plato's dialogue *Cratylus*.

In the case of this book, an exhaustive definition of the key concepts that make up the theme of the book, namely human reproductive cloning, uniqueness, and dignity, would be impossible for several reasons: First, I am not a geneticist or biologist, so it would be very risky to seek a concise definition of human cloning. Therefore, in what follows, I will only attempt to convey to the reader what I understand human cloning to be after reviewing the relevant literature. Second, both the concept of uniqueness and that of dignity are extremely challenging, rich, and ambiguous. It takes more than a few pages to even begin to outline either concept. In fact, much

---

[1] Antisthenis, *Fragmenta*, ed. Fernanda Decleva Caizzi (Milano, and Varese: Instituto Editoriale Cisalpino, 1965), D38: "The beginning of education is the definition of terms." The fragment is mentioned in Epictetus' *Discourses* – see next note.

[2] Epictetus, *Discourses of Epictetus*, trans. George Long (New York: D. Appleton and Co., 1904), Book I, XVII.

ink has been spent over the centuries trying to understand these concepts, so far without much success. In view of this, I had no choice but to propose the approach or approaches that I believe would be more fruitful for discussing the subject of this book, human reproductive cloning.

I. Cloning: What, how, why, and why not

It is often said that art copies nature; well, science also does so, and cloning is an iconic case of copying nature. Even first-year biology students are aware of the fact that with regard to the plant kingdom the existence of genetically identical organisms is a common phenomenon – so common that we do not even use the term 'clones,' but 'varieties' instead. When it comes to animal species, the presence of identical copies is much rarer. In several cases, however, such as in the case of single-celled protozoa like amoebae or bacteria, for example, reproduction takes place by means of binary fission, a process that produces two individuals with identical genomes,[3] a process that could accurately be described as cloning.[4] Some invertebrates also have the ability to regenerate fully as complete organisms from a small original part of theirs. Vertebrates lack this ability, but to some extent some of them can regenerate tissues, limbs, and organs.[5] It is statistically rare, but it is still a probability in

[3] See James Young Simpson, "The Relation of Binary Fission to Variation," *Biometrika* 1, no. 4 (1902): 402; also, Herbert Spencer Jennings, "Heredity, Variation and Evolution in Protozoa II. Heredity and Variation of Size and Form in Paramecium, with Studies of Growth, Environmental Action and Selection," *Proceedings of the American Philosophical Society* 47, no. 190 (1908): 393-546.

[4] David N. Wells, "Animal Cloning: Problems and Prospects," *Scientific and Technical Review of the Office International des Epizooties* 24, no. 1 (2005): 251.

[5] National Bioethics Advisory Commission, *Cloning Human Beings: Report*

the case of higher mammals that the division of a fertilized egg would result to two identical individuals, each one having the same genotype and phenotype as the other: This is the case of homozygous twins.[6]

Although to a large extent replication is a natural process that facilitates reproduction on a species level on the one hand, and also regeneration on individual level on the other, when it comes to human reproductive cloning, as it is always the case when natural *randomness* (or, necessity) is attempted to be artificially imitated and applied, an abundance of serious ethical questions and dilemmas arise, questions and dilemmas that fuel one among the most heated ethical debates of our times, the one on human reproductive cloning.

Cloning, though, is neither primarily, nor mainly, aimed at the replication of human individuals; as a matter of fact, human reproductive cloning is but a small cluster of a much broader scientific field, ranging from single-cell replication to the creation of identical organisms, and, as far as the latter is concerned, not always aiming to reproduction. As a generic procedure cloning is defined as the process of artificially (that is, under laboratory conditions) generating an exact (identical) genetic copy (called the *clone*) of any kind of biological material (called the *prototype*), be it a piece of DNA, a molecule, an individual cell, a plant, an animal, or a full human being. At the same time, the term also designates the scientific

---

and Recommendations (Rockville, MD, 1997), 14.

[6] Mario F. Fraga, et al., "Epigenetic Differences Arise During the Lifetime of Monozygotic Twins," *Proceedings of the National Academy of Sciences* 102, no. 30 (2005): 10604. More recent research, however, questions the genotypic identity of homozygous twins; see Carl E. G. Bruder, et al., "Phenotypically Concordant and Discordant Monozygotic Twins Display Different DNA Copy-Number-Variation Profiles," *The American Journal of Human Genetics* 82, no. 3 (2008): 768ff.

research field that investigates and applies particular technologies, and nowadays constitutes an important subfield of experimental biology.[7]

a. From a frog to a sheep

In mammals, including humans, the method that has proved most successful so far is somatic cell nuclear transfer, and it has been the advances in this procedure that have brought the possibility of asexual reproduction in humans within reach: And this, even if it remains for the moment only a prospect, is definitely the culmination of a relatively short but rather glorious scientific journey. The description that follows provides a good overview of the potential, but also the limitations of cloning via somatic cell nuclear transfer:

> Cloning is achieved by somatic cell nuclear transfer (SCNT), in which chromosomes are first removed from an egg to create an enucleated egg. The chromosomes are then replaced with a nucleus derived from a somatic cell of the individual or embryo to be cloned.[8] Factors in the cytoplasm of the enucleated oocyte cause "reprogramming" or de-differentiation of the transferred nucleus so that it regains the full developmental potential of a zygotic (fertilized) nucleus, as occurs in the usual fusion of egg and

---

[7] National Bioethics Advisory Commission, *Cloning Human Beings: Report and Recommendations of the National Bioethics Advisory Commission* (Rockville, MD, 1997), 13.

[8] As cited in Malby, see below. R. S. Prather, and N. L. First, "Cloning of Embryos," *Journal of Reproduction and Fertility Supplment* 40 (1990): 227-234.

sperm.[9] However, the construct created by SCNT also contains small amounts of extra-nuclear DNA derived from the egg (mtDNA).[10] Strictly speaking, therefore, a cloned person would not be 100% genetically identical to the prototype, since they would not have the same mtDNA (unless the female donor were to clone herself and also use one of her own eggs).[11]

Nevertheless, somatic cell nuclear transfer, the best possibility available to us today to reproduce identical copies of humans asexually, did not appear out of nowhere. The relatively short history of cloning began in the late 19th century with a frog and culminated in the present day with a sheep.

In 1892 the German evolutionary biologist August Weismann published his work *Das Germplasm: Eine Theorie der Vererbung*,[12] which he dedicated to the memory of Charles Darwin. In it he articulated for the first time his *germ plasm theory*: He argued, in particular, that multicellular organisms are composed of *germ cells* (gametes, that is, eggs and sperm cells) on the one hand, cells that contain inherited genetic information, and *somatic cells* on the other, whose purpose is to form organs, bones and tissue, and perform somatic functions; he also realized that inheritance may take place only through

[9] As cited in Malby, see below. M. Munsie, C. O'brien, and P. Mountford, "Transgenic Strategy for Demonstrating Nuclear Reprogramming in the Mouse," *Cloning Stem Cells* 4, no. 2 (2002): 121-130.

[10] As cited in Malby, see below. M. J. Evans et al., "Mitochondrial DNA Genotypes in Nuclear Transfer- derived Cloned Sheep," *Nature Genetics* 23, no. 1 (1999): 90-93.

[11] Steven Malby, "Human Dignity and Human Reproductive Cloning," *Health and Human Rights* 6, no. 1 (2002): 105.

[12] August Weismann, *Das Germplasm: Eine Theorie der Vererbung* (Jena: Fischer, 1982).

germ cells, but not through somatic cells. And while the latter are subject to environmental or other influences during
the organism's lifetime, germ cells remain unchanged and are
passed on intact to the organism's offspring. Sperm cells divide to produce somatic cells, which, however, do not possess
all the genetic material of the original cell, but only that which
is necessary for them to perform specialized functions. In other words, pancreatic cells may be the outcome of several successive divisions of a single germ cell, but they lack a large part
of the genetic information contained in the initial germ cell.
The information contained in them cannot be passed on to
the offspring of the organism, since the transfer of genetic fea-
tures is only achieved through germ cells. Hence, contrary to
what Lamarck had assumed,[13] Weismann maintained that acquired characteristics cannot be inherited.[14] Weismann's views
found enormous support in the findings of Wilhelm Roux, a
German zoologist experimental researcher who, after having
used a red-hot needle to destroy one of the two blastomeres of
the embryo of a frog belonging to the species *Rana fusca*, observed that the remaining cell developed into an incomplete
embryo; to him this was a proof that, already at the stage of the
initial division, the original cell had lost half of the complete
genetic information it originally contained.[15]

---

[13] Jean-Baptiste Lamarck maintains that acquired characteristics can be
transmitted to the offspring of an organism through propagation; see among
others Richard W. Burkhardt, Jr., "Lamarck, Evolution, and the Inheritance
of Acquired Characters," *Genetics* 194, no. 4 (2013): 793-805.

[14] See August Weismann, *The Germ-Plasm: A Theory of Heredity*, trans. W.
Newton Parker, and Harriet Rönnfeldt (New York: Charles Scribner's Sons,
1898; reprinted by Nabu Press, 2010), especially 450ff.

[15] The experiment and Roux's findings were published in 1988 as "Über
die künstliche Hervorbringung halber Embryonen durch Zerstörung
einer der beiden ersten Furchungszellen, sowie über die Nachtentwicklung
(Postgeneration) der fehltenden Körperhälfte," *Virchows Archive für*

Weismann's theory of cellular specialization was chal-lenged by the German biologist and philosopher Hans Dri-esch in 1891. Driesch was able to demonstrate experimentally that the blastomeres of a sea urchin embryo can develop into complete organisms at the stage of division of the original cell into 2 and 4 cells. Thus, the division of the original embryonic cell does not result in a reduction of the original genetic in-formation: When the cells resulting from the division of the original cell are uncoupled and isolated, each of them in turn begins to divide, retaining the ability to develop into any cell type, just like the original *totipotent* cell.[16] The fact that Dri-esch succeeded in separating the two blastomeres and produc-ing two identical organisms from them is often regarded as the first case of successful cloning of a multicellular organism.[17]

A few years later, in 1901, the German embryologist Hans Spemann, who later received the Nobel Prize, confirmed the results of Driesch's research.[18] Spemann used a strand of his daughter's hair to form a loop with which he divided a sala-mander embryo into two parts: One in which the nucleus of the embryo was enclosed, and another in which only cyto-plasm and other cellular material remained. One side of the nucleus began to dissolve, but the other side did not. When the embryo had already divided four times and reached the stage of dividing into 16 cells, Spemann loosened the loop so

---

Pathologische Anatomie und Physiologie 114 (1988): 419-521.

[16] Hans Driesch, "Entwicklungsmechanisme Studien. I. Der Werth der beiden ersten Furchungszellen in der Echinodermentwicklung. Experimentelle Erzeugung von Theil und Doppelbildungen," *Zeitschrift für wissenschaftliche Zoologie* 53 (1891): 160-184.

[17] Michael Bellomo, *The Stem Cell Divide: The Facts, the Fiction, And the Fear Driving the Greatest Scientific, Political and Religious Debate of Our Time* (New York: AMACOM, 2006), 134.

[18] See Hans Spemann, *Embryo Development and Induction* (New Haven, CT: Yale University Press, 1938).

that one of the sixteen cells could be transferred to the immature part, where the division process began immediately. Spemann then separated the two embryos and allowed them to develop into two identical twin salamanders.[19] Spemann's success was the precursor to cloning by nuclear transfer, a technique now widely used in animal cloning and therapeutic cloning research.[20]

Following Spemann's example, biologists Robert Briggs and Thomas King succeeded in transferring the nucleus of an adult frog cell into a *naked egg*, thus producing the first clone in 1952. Six years later, British molecular biologist John Gurdon definitively disproved Weismann's theory that it is impossible to produce clones from differentiated cells because the specialized cells of adult organisms have lost some of their original genetic material. Gurdon created thirty clones of Xenopus frogs by transferring the nucleus from somatic cells of a tadpole with albinism into immature tadpole eggs with the usual coloration for the species. The clones, of course, were not white. Gurdon's success proved that even in differentiated, specialized cells, the genome remains unchanged.[21] His experiments also provided the impetus for the recognition of cloning as a new scientific possibility: In 1963, the British biologist John Burdon Haldane used the term *clone* for animals, which until then had been used only in reference to plants.[22] Things were now well underway.

---

[19] Ryuzo Yanagimachi, "Cloning: Experience from the Mouse and Other Animals," *Molecular and Cellular Endocrinology* 187 (2002): 241.

[20] Xavier Vignon, Yvan Heyman, P. Chavatte-Palmer, and J. P. Renard, "Biotechnologies de la reproduction: le clonage des animaux d'élevage," *Inra Production Animales* 21, no. 1 (2008): 34.

[21] Jane Maienschein, *Whose View of Life? Embryos, Cloning, and Stem Cells* (New York: Harvard University Press, 2003), 122ff.

[22] Haldane's talk "Biological Possibilities for the Human Species in the

In 1995, cloning went from the stage of possibility to that of reality: Ian Wilmut and Keith Campbell, both biologists at the Roslin Institute in Edinburgh, Scotland, successfully cloned two sheep, Megan and Morag, using cells they had taken from differentiated embryos and placed in an egg from which they had removed the genetic material. However, this was only the prelude to what was to follow next year: The same scientists managed to create the first clone from adult somatic cells, demonstrating what the scientific community had been preparing for almost a century. Sheep No. 6LL3, which was given the name 'Dolly,' was created by introducing the nucleus from a mature, differentiated cell from the mammary gland of an adult sheep into an enucleated egg cell.[23]

The birth of 'Dolly' turned the previously established biological facts completely upside down, namely the assumption that it is impossible to recreate a whole cell with complete genetic material from the original cell once it has differentiated into fully specialized organ and tissue cells. Dolly the sheep lived only six years, far less than the survival expectation of her species describes. She developed a lung tumor and showed early symptoms of arthritis. Many researchers attribute this to the fact that she was created from a cell that was already six years old and therefore afflicted with the degenerative effects of time.[24] This suspicion has never been substantiated and remains in abeyance to this day. The success of Wilmut and Campbell's experiment, however, is in no way diminished by this. For what their experiment proved in the first place was

Next Ten Thousand Years" is included in *Man and His Future*, ed. Gordon Wolstenholme, 337-361 (Boston: Little, Brown and Company, 1963).

[23] Ian Wilmut, et al., "Viable Offspring Derived from Fetal and Adult Mammalian Cells," *Nature* 385 (1997): 810-813.

[24] J. Giles, and J. Knight, "Dolly's Death Leaves Researchers Woolly on Clone Ageing Issue," *Nature* 421 (2003): 776.

that the course of cellular differentiation and specialization is reversible. This finding was enough to trigger a revolution in biology and genetics that heralded the beginning of a wondrous new world. Such a nuclear transfer experiment was also performed with an enucleated human oocyte and the nucleus of an adult human skin cell.[25] The construct was not implanted, but was only allowed to develop (apparently normally) to the six-cell stage before being destroyed.[26]

b. Not just sci-fi extravaganza

People's imagination is always captured by the extravagant and the spectacular, usually to the detriment of what is valuable but not captivating – and cloning is no exception to the rule. Nevertheless, and despite the fact that public attention is, as expected, almost exclusively fixated on the potential cloning of human beings, cloning is not only that, and not even primarily that: On the contrary, its actual and potential applications cover an extremely broad spectrum. Molecular biologists and geneticists today are capable of cloning DNA fragments and sequences, cell lines, and entire organisms. In the first case, parts of the DNA sequence are copied and inserted into a host cell, usually a bacterium. Bacteria are prokaryotic organisms, which means that they do not have an organized nucleus. This allows them to multiply extremely rapidly by simple branching, resulting in identical organisms. So, the original bacterium, into which scientists have inserted part of a DNA sequence, when bred, can produce hundreds of identical parts of the original sequence in a very short time, expanding experimental possibilities.

[25] J. B. Cibelli, et al., "Somatic Cell Nuclear Transfer in Humans: Pronuclear and Early Embryonic Development," *e-biomed: The Journal of Regenerative Medicine* 2 (2001): 25-31.

[26] Malby, 108.

Molecular cloning has been used for decades for experimental purposes, with brilliant results: As early as 1980, diabetes was treated by administering insulin (rHI) produced thanks to DNA recombination in bacterial lines,[27] while anemia is treated by administration of recombinant erythropoietin (r-HuEPO), which is also the result of molecular cloning.[28]

Cell and cell-line cloning is also performed for experimental therapeutic purposes and the development of pharmaceutical substances. In this context somatic cells are removed from an organism and cultured under laboratory conditions to produce cell lines identical to those of the donor. The cloned cells are then used to test new drugs on them.[29] Preclinical in vitro screening on cloned cells and cell-lines is essential to assess the efficacy of compounds before they enter the initial preclinical phase of animal testing, as this can significantly reduce costs and accelerate the development of certain drugs. On the other hand, the recent establishment of stem cells in various tissues has opened new horizons for studies that are based on cell cloning, as this allows researchers to study cell self-renewal and multipotency in a variety of identical samples. Stem cell cloning opens up new opportunities for biologists and geneticists to unravel the mechanisms of organ regeneration, and brings closer the prospect of making organ transplantation obsolete – fulfilling thus the wishes of millions of people on transplant lists around the world.

The cloning of whole organisms – I mean here: of animals and, especially, of mammals – aims at creating identical indi-

---

[27] See Arthur Riggs, "Bacterial Production of Human Insulin," *Diabetes Care* 4, no. 1 (1981): 64-68.

[28] See Joan C. Egrie, "The Cloning and Production of Recombinant Human Erythropoietin," *Pharmacotherapy* 10, no. 2 (1990): 3S-8S.

[29] National Bioethics Advisory Commission, *Cloning Human Beings: Report and Recommendations* (Rockville, MD, 1997), 14.

viduals of any species. As shown above, this is done either by separating the blastomeres, or by removing the nucleus from a single cell, either somatic or stem cell, and reintroducing it into another stem or somatic cell, from which the original nucleus has been removed.[30] The motivation for mammalian cloning is twofold: On the one hand it is the basic *scientific curiosity* that has driven human science since its inception, and on the other hand it is a *necessity*, but not always *so* basic: In addition to creating individuals to be used for biotechnological studies, as in the cloning of cells and cell lines, contemporary science seems also to entertain much broader aspirations: Somatic cell nuclear transfer makes it possible to produce identical animals so as to preserve endangered species,[31] and even to restore extinct species by harvesting fossilized genetic material (somatic cells), and then inserting it into enucleated egg cells extracted from individuals of closely related species that exist in the present.[32] *De-extinction*, in particular, the prospect of 'resurrecting' long-extinct species and make extinction "no longer forever,"[33] is a fascinating prospect indeed, and by all means equally challenging for ethics. In a profound and groundbreaking essay of his, Shlomo Cohen discusses five dimensions that cut across the ethical implications of reviving extinct species, namely:

---

[30] Ibid., 15-16.

[31] The prospect is often referred to as 'de-extinction.' See among others Kenneth Lee, "Can Cloning Save Endangered Species?" *Current Biology* 11, no. 7 (2001): R245-R246.

[32] See among various others Beth Shapiro, "Pathways to De-extinction: How Close Can We Get to Resurrection of an Extinct Species?" *Functional Ecology* 31, no. 5 (2017): 996-1002.

[33] George Church, Ed Regis, *Regenesis: How Synthetic Biology Will Reinvent Nature and Ourselves* (New York: Basic Books, 2012).

the axiological question of promoting ecological values, the deontological question of whether we owe de-extinction to species we rendered extinct, the ethical-existential question of "playing God" through de-extinction, the utilitarian perspective, and the place of aesthetic considerations in the ethics of de-extinction.[34]

Yet, applying somatic cell cloning on animals for the purpose of bringing species that no longer exist back to life in order to restore the injustice inflicted upon them by our species in the past, or to increase bio-diversity for the benefit of existing people, future generations, and life on earth in general, is again just what catches the eye; there are still some much more practical and less controversial uses of cloning in animals.

Mammalian cloning, for instance, may also aim not at generating live animals, but instead creating "genetically matched, immunologically compatible (autologous) stem cells that can potentially differentiate in such a way as to replace damaged or diseased tissues or organs in an adult,"[35] or facilitating the treatment of various diseases – in both non-human and human animals. Cloning animal stem-cells – which do not necessarily have to be derived from animal embryos – also has the potential to reduce the number of laboratory animals: Immunologically compatible tissues could be produced, on which researchers could test substances instead of testing them on live animals directly. For some this is also a response to the most common accusation against animal

---

[34] Shlomo Cohen, "The Ethics of De-Extinction," *Nanoethics* 8 (2014): 166

[35] Anna-Katerina Hadjantonakis, and Virginia E Papaioannou, "Can Mammalian Cloning Combined with Embryonic Stem Cell Technologies Be Used to Treat Human Diseases?" *Genome Biology* 3, no. 8 (2002): 1023.1-1023.6.

cloning, namely that it is primarily aimed at human ends. It is not necessarily untrue that "some animal cloning projects are motivated by regard or concern for animals as ends in themselves"[36] by seeking to create disease-resistant animals, and thus increase animal welfare.

Of these three applications of cloning (of molecules, cell lines, and full organisms), the last, especially mammalian cloning, is understandably the one that has been most criticized and has raised persistent ethical concerns, primarily because it anticipates the possibility of reproductive cloning of humans. In addition to concerns based on uniqueness and dignity, on which this book will focus exclusively, there are also concerns about the efficiency of whole-organisms cloning in producing viable offspring. But the cloning of cells and cell lines is not free of ethical concerns either, especially when human embryonic stem cells are involved: Omnipotent embryonic stem cells have the potential to develop into a fetus and a human being, and this makes their destruction during cloning ethically controversial: To many this seems to violate the beginning of human life and personhood.

Depending on the purpose it serves, cloning is also classified as therapeutic or reproductive. However, this distinction is often considered irrelevant or superfluous, as there is no clear dividing line between these two types.[37] Therapeutic cloning usually refers to the duplication of stem cells for ex-

---

[36] Autumn Fiester, "Ethical Issues in Animal Cloning," *Perspectives in Biology and Medicine* 48, no. 3 (2005): 330.

[37] The term *reproductive* cloning is actually a platitude, since cloning is by definition a reproductive process. See John Finnis, "Some Fundamental Evils in Generating Human Embryos by Cloning," in *Ethics and Law in Biological Research*, ed. Cosimo Marco Mazzoni, 99-106 (The Hague: Kluwer, 2002), 100: "[…] a vocabulary was devised and popularized according to which there are two kinds of cloning to produce human embryos, […] therapeutic and […] reproductive. This vocabulary should be rejected as politicized and

perimental or therapeutic purposes, or to the creation of embryos for the production of embryonic stem cells whose DNA will be identical to that of the donor – although the latter, as I mentioned earlier, is highly controversial and strictly prohibited[38]: The main problem (for some, *the only* one) consists in that the harvesting of cloned stem cells inevitably leads to the destruction of the embryo produced. Despite the controversies that still exist, therapeutic cloning is quite promising in terms of tissue (and organ) regeneration and *de novo* organ synthesis.[39]

Reproductive cloning, on the other hand, distinguishes between human cloning and cloning of nonhuman mammals, as described in previous sections, the first type being ethically controversial, the second not – or at least not so much. The prospect of preserving endangered species, even recovering lost ones, and propagating rare breeds, is balanced against the dangers associated with the production of crossbred or transgenic animals, whether for livestock farming, or simply to create unnecessary and, at the end of the day, unwanted biodiversity.[40]

---

manipulative. Production of embryos by cloning is always reproductive, for it is always and necessarily reproduction – generation of one human being from another – even when the further aim is that the embryo so produced shall later be destroyed rather than proceed to independent life as a breathing child." However, given the fact that the term has been established in the relevant literature. See for example Chamundeeswari Kuppuswamy, et al., *Is Human Reproductive Cloning Inevitable: Future Options for UN Governance* (Yokohama: United States University – Institute for Advanced Studies, 1997), I will use it for the sake of consistency and compatibility.

[38] The Oviedo Convention, for instance, stipulates that "the creation of human embryos for research is prohibited."

[39] Charlotte Kfoury, "Therapeutic Cloning: Promises and Issues," *McGill Journal of Medicine* 10, no. 2 (2007): 113.

[40] Lawrence C. Smith, Vilceu Bordignon, Marie Babkine, Gilles Fecteau, and

c. New prospects, new challenges

I cannot think of any scientific achievement, innovation, or technological advance that didn't first emerge amidst a host of moral concerns and ethical challenges. The most telling example is by far in vitro fertilization, the last scientific breakthrough before cloning, which was certainly greeted with great hopes, but it was also met with the greatest fears and ethical reservations: Overcoming natural conception, transcending the limits of the human body by post-menopause propagation, creating "human monsters"[41] and doing "the devil's work,"[42] these and other arguments as such eventually proved to be no match for the hopes of thousands of couples with fertility problems. But even after decades since it was first introduced into clinical practice, and after the birth of more than ten million people thanks to this method, the ethical debate about in vitro fertilization is still heated, even if it is now moving in other directions. It couldn't be different in the case of cloning, especially since its potential seems to anticipate the asexual reproduction of human beings.

As I mentioned earlier, no type of cloning is unassailable to ethical criticism. Even animal cloning, which might seem to some to be the least ethically problematic kind, is accompanied by moral concerns related to the potentially negative consequences for, and the dangers to animal and human health and welfare, as well as the stability and balance of the environment. What adds to these concerns is that somatic

Carol Keefer, "Benefits and Problems with Cloning Animals," *The Canadian Veterinary Journal* 41 (2000): 919-924.

[41] M. Mulkay, "Frankenstein and the Debate over Embryo Research," *Science, Technology and Human Values* 21, no. 2 (1996): 157-176.

[42] Reinhold Manhart, "Medizin-Nobelpreis für ein Teufelswerk," *MMW – Fortschritte der Medizin* 152, no. 41 (2010): 6.

cell nuclear transfer, when applied to animals, brings even closer the creation of *chimeras*, i.e., animal embryos with different cell populations derived from more than one species: Already cases have been reported of viable mouse-rat chimeric embryos that have been created by means of embryonic stem cell microinjection;[43] somatic cell nuclear transfer, however, combined with genetic engineering opens new horizons for science: It might not be long before human-animal chimeras could be created,[44] or human organs could be 'cultivated' in chimeric animals.[45] All of these, and other issues as such, raise numerous ethical questions about animal cloning. In my view, however, these concerns are only the visible tip of the iceberg. The real fear that hides beneath the surface is that animal cloning could become the 'thin edge of the wedge' that would inevitably lead to the gradual devaluation – and eventual violation – of crucial prohibitions and fundamental principles, paving thus the way for human reproductive cloning as well.[46]

Cloning of single cells and tissues is also fraught with ethical concerns. In particular, therapeutic embryonic stem cell research raises a number of ethical and legal issues, ranging from the moral and legal status of the embryo and, con-

---

[43] Barbara K. Stepien, Samir Vaid, Ronald Naumann, Anja Holtz, and Wieland B. Huttner, "Generation of Interspecies Mouse-rat Chimeric Embryos by Embryonic Stem (ES) Cell Microinjection," *Protocols* 2 (2021): 100494; also Davor Solter, "Viable Rat-Mouse Chimeras: Where Do We Go from Here?" *Cell* 142 (2010): 676-678.

[44] Victoria L. Mascetti, and Roger A. Pedersen, "Human-monkey Chimeras: Monkey See, Monkey Do," *Cell Stem Cell* 28 (2021): 787-789.

[45] Yingfei Lu, Yu Zhou, Rong Ju, and Jianquan Chen, "Human-animal Chimeras for Autologous Organ Transplantation: Technological Advances and Future Perspectives," *Annals of Translational Medicine* 7, no. 20 (2019): 576-584.

[46] See Fiester, 330.

sequently, the moral permissibility of destroying the blasto-cyst so as to obtain stem cells,[47] to the intentional creation of spare embryos to serve as fields for the cultivation of single cells or organs.[48] Single cell and tissue cloning is classified as 'therapeutic,' and is by and large permitted by all inter-national conventions, while at the same time "the creation of human embryos for research is prohibited."[49] However, to the extent that research regards omnipotent cells, usually 'spare' embryos should be cloned; that is, both therapeutic and reproductive cloning depend on the in vitro generation of human embryos, thus "prohibiting reproductive cloning is likely to result in severely hindering medically important research based on therapeutic cloning."[50] As promising as therapeutic cloning may be for humanity, it seems that it is largely impossible to reap its benefits without first allowing at least some forms of reproductive cloning.

The question is, and this one is a philosophical ques-tion indeed, where we should draw the line of demarcation between reproductive and therapeutic cloning. As things stand, the science and technology that is available to date could only support cloning of human organisms by nuclear transfer. In this technique, the nucleus of a mature human somatic cell is removed and inserted into an enucleated fe-male human germ cell (egg cell) ready to receive the nucleus of the donor. The egg cell is then subjected to electrical puls-

---

[47] The literature is vast; see among others Bernard Lo, and Lindsay Parham, "Ethical Issues in Stem Cell Research," *Endocrine Reviews* 30, no. 3 (2009): 204-213.

[48] Michael J. Sandel, "The Ethical Implications of Human Cloning," *Perspectives in Biology and Medicine* 48, no. 2 (2005): 244ff.

[49] *The Oviedo Convention*, article 18.

[50] Kfoury, 113.

es and begins to divide until it reaches the blastocyst stage,[51] and is ready for implantation in the endometrium. If the normal process of successive divisions continues even there, an embryo will be formed which can be born normally, giving rise to the clone of the individual from whose body cell the nucleus was originally taken. It is plain that the whole process of cloning is divided into two phases: the preparation phase (removal of the nucleus from the recipient oocyte, extraction of the nucleus from the donor somatic cell, introduction of the nucleus into the recipient oocyte, genetic programming of the oocyte), and the implantation phase.[52] To be able to speak properly of human reproductive cloning – or attempted cloning – the second stage should be also completed, that is, "the resulting human embryo is implanted and develops to full term."[53] This seems to imply that the creation of an early embryo that would be artificially created, but it would not be allowed to develop beyond a certain stage, and in no case be carried to term, would not fall under the category of reproductive cloning. However, this approach would be in deep conflict with some deeply entrenched onto-logical, metaphysical, and religious views: To many 'reproduc-tion' has already been completed in conception, and the view that it hasn't fails to see that "Human embryos are not potential persons; they are actual persons with potential."[54] It is true that

---

[51] The blastocyst begins to form on the fifth day. Implantation into the mitochondrion is possible even earlier when the oocyte into which the donor nucleus was introduced is at the stage of the morsel. However, blastocyst implantation is considered to be much more effective. See Michelle Plachot, "The Blastocyst," *Human Reproduction* 15, no. 4 (2000): 49.

[52] Since "Federal authority can make it illegal to implant a cloned embryo into a uterus;" see Raymond Barglow, "Therapeutic Cloning Can Save Lives," in *The Ethics of Human Cloning*, ed. John Woodward, 30-36 (Farmington Hills, MI: Thomson Gale, 2005), 35.

[53] Malby, 105.

[54] Clinton Wilcox, "The Human Embryo: Potential Person or Person with

the argument from potentiality has attracted severe criticism even among distinguished theologians. Dunstan has famously supported the view that,

> the claim to absolute protection for the human embryo 'from the beginning' is a novelty in the Western, Christian and specifically Roman Catholic moral traditions. It is virtually a creation of the later nineteenth century, a little over a century ago; and that is a novelty indeed as traditions go.[55]

Dunstan bases his assertion on the relevant views of various scholars, philosophers, and religious figures, from Aristotle to St Basil the Great, St Thomas Aquinas and John de Lugo. The fact remains, however: Delayed ensoulment is not the dominant current in Christian theology,[56] and this, of course, has significant implications for the moral and ontological status ascribed to embryos. From this perspective the cloning of embryos – even if they are not intended to be born, but only to be used for research purposes – is always reproductive and therefore morally reprehensible – and also legally unacceptable.

d. A sign of coming to age – and some thoughts on moral and human rights

Given that human reproductive cloning is today at best a possibility, but not a tangible reality – as no human organism has

---

Great Potential?" *Christian Research Journal* 40, no. 3 (2017): 1.

[55] Gordon Reginald Dunstan, "The Moral Status of the Human Embryo: A Tradition Recalled," *Journal of Medical Ethics* 1 (1984): 38.

[56] For a fierce polemic against Dunstan views see among others D. A. Jones, "The Human Embryo in the Christian Tradition: A Reconsideration," *Journal of Medical Ethics* 31 (2005): 710-714.

yet been demonstrably cloned[57] – the ethical debate over cloning is one of the few fortunate occasions when ethics – in this case, bioethics – can deal in advance with, rather than hurry after, a burning ethical issue. Unlike, for example, the use of nuclear energy for peaceful purposes or the production of genetically modified foods, in the case of human cloning bioethics has been given both the opportunity, as well as a seemingly reasonable time, to evaluate the possibilities and draw conclusions. Under all possible aspects, this is definitely a sign of the very much needed and overwhelmingly belated moral maturity of our species.

And while this is good news for our species, and also good fortune for bioethics – and a rare one, it is nevertheless accompanied by seriously troubling consequences: Precisely because human cloning has not yet moved from the stage of possibility to that of reality, the relevant ethical debate can only be largely speculative, that is, it runs the risk of focusing on parameters that may be overridden by scientific developments. Moreover, precisely because of the early stage at which the technological possibility of human cloning is at, it is reasonable and therefore justifiable that the relevant arguments for and against this possibility be laden with hopes and suspicions that are likely to prove unfounded in the future.

The main ethical considerations about human reproductive cloning revolve around two main axes: One focuses on the rights of human individuals, while the other explores the potential benefits and harms that human cloning may bring to both the clone and the prototype, as well as to human soci-

---

[57] Among biologists there is huge and ever-growing skepticism about the possibility of successfully cloning not just human beings, but even primates; for a brief but very informative outline of these concerns see Philip Cohen, "Cloning Humans May Be Impossible," in *The Ethics of Human Cloning*, ed. John Woodward, 54-56 (Farmington Hills, MI: Thomson Gale, 2005).

eties and the species. As for the first axis, cloning is discussed in terms of human dignity. This inevitably directs the debate to the discussion of the human and moral rights that seem to be at risk at the prospect of human reproductive cloning. The second axis clearly has a consequentialist orientation. In what follows, I will focus on the first group of concerns, i.e., the extent to which human reproductive cloning might preserve or endanger human dignity and rights.

At this point, I must clarify that, although I have spoken above of moral *and* human rights, I do not consider human rights as sharply distinct from moral rights, but rather as a subset of them; I fully endorse the view that "human rights are moral rights that people have because of their membership in the human family, not because of any external force or agency;"[58] but the way I understand the phrase 'because of their membership in the human family' is probably not exactly what one would expect: In my view belonging to the human family means being endowed with certain intellectual capacities, by virtue of which the very notion of human rights – as well as certain human rights – is *conceivable*, and *justifiable* as "a class of moral consideration whose only role in political discourse is to justify coercive intervention in a society's affairs."[59] Whether it is rationality, as Immanuel Kant suggests, or a sense of *decency*, as John Rawls assumes,[60] or anything else, to be a member of the human family in my view is to be able to detach one's self from the particular circumstances surrounding one's existence, and

---

[58] Dominic Stolerman, "The Moral Foundations of Human Rights Attitudes," *Political Psychology* 41, no. 3 (2020): 439; see also J. Morsink, *The Universal Declaration of Human Rights: Origins, Drafting, and Intent* (Philadelphia: University of Pennsylvania Press, 1999), 208.

[59] Charles R. Beitz, "Human Rights as a Common Concern," *American Political Science Review* 95, no. 2 (2001): 276.

[60] John Rawls introduces the rather ambiguous notion of 'decency' in his

to recognize on moral – rather than empirical – grounds that every human being *should be* allowed this or that freedom just because it is a human being – not because human beings are by their nature *capable of* enjoying this or that particular freedom, but because *there are good moral reasons* why one should enjoy such a freedom, and also good moral reasons why one should not be prevented from enjoying that freedom.

I must admit that this approach of mine presupposes a profoundly optimistic view of the powers of the human intellect, a view that may seem to some to be entirely arbitrary: That humans are capable of using their intellectual powers in such a way as to distance themselves from the reality they experience, judge it *in abstracto* on moral grounds, and if necessary, reject it in favor of another reality that would be more reasonable, or more descent, or morally justifiable. This means, for example, that the members of a society in which the practice of clitoridectomy is interwoven with the local culture, and has been performed continuously over the years, might nevertheless upon proper reflection abandon that practice on the grounds that women are being used merely as a means, and not at the same time as an end in themselves, which is utterly irrational and self-defeating. This could also apply to the hypothetical case of women who would be willing – or even eager – to have their own clitoris removed in order to enjoy higher social status, find a husband more easily, and so on: They would treat their own self merely as a means to an end, and that, in turn, would be completely irrational and self-defeating.

It is true that my approach endures to the extent that the powers of the human intellect for abstract meditation are in-

"The Law of Peoples," *Critical Inquiry* 20, no. 1 (1993): 36-68, by referring to 'decent governments' and 'decent societies,' and maintaining that "insisting on human rights is exerting pressure in the direction of decent governments and a decent society of peoples;" see 65, n. 52.

deed so strong; but I also feel that the whole structure of ethics can endure only to the same extent. On the other hand, this approach easily escapes the 'is-ought' fallacy, of which views of natural rights are so often accused. For example, instead of asserting that "Women should be entitled to keep their clitoris, because by their nature women *do* have a clitoris, and *are* also *inclined* to keep it," this approach assumes that "Women should be entitled to keep their clitoris, because by their nature all people upon proper reflection can understand that there are good moral reasons in favor of this, and none at all in favor of the opposite;" in other words, that it is absolutely rational to affirm the former, while it is absolutely irrational to affirm the latter.

Thus, human rights may be conceivable as moral guidelines or, even, imperatives that depend on the common intellectual heritage of the species *Homo sapiens*, that is, the intellectual capacities and strengths that all human beings have 'because of their membership in the human family,' rather than on their actual capacities, inclinations, or condition. In this sense, human rights are political instruments that are supported by moral arguments and justification. In the words of Charles Beitz,

> the doctrine of human rights is a political construction intended for certain political purposes and is to be understood against the background of a range of general assumptions about the character of the contemporary international environment [...] as principles for international affairs that could be accepted by reasonable persons who hold conflicting reasonable conceptions of the good life.[61]

---

[61] Beitz, "Human Rights as a Common Concern," 276.

To sum up, the fact that I refer to moral *and* human rights is not aimed at distinguishing one from the other in terms of content or justification, but at emphasizing the specificity of human rights in terms of their function as political instruments. My view is that, unlike common – or, standard – moral rights, once each right that belongs to this special category has been established, then it becomes legally binding by virtue of the treaty in which it is enshrined, so that its beneficiaries can invoke and claim it before state and transnational institutions and authorities, which is not the case with common moral rights.

II. Bioethics, and why it is relevant

In April 1985, the then President of the French Republic, François Mitterrand, in his opening speech at an international bioethics conference in Rambouillet, among other things claimed:

> At its heart, the history of human rights, which rightly provokes so much controversy, is the history of a conquest: the idea of man. What will happen now if this concept of man can be modified by science? What will happen to concepts as fundamental as life, death, kinship?[62]

---

[62] "L'examen des projets sur la bioéthique Commentaire La loi et les mœurs," *Le Monde*, January 14, 1994, https://www.lemonde.fr/archives/article/1994/01/14/l-examen-des-projets-sur-la-bioethique-commentaire-la-loi-et-les-moeurs_3798293_1819218.html: "au fond, l'histoire des droits de l'homme, qui suscite à juste titre tant de passions, c'est l'histoire d'une conquête, l'idée de personne humaine. Que faire alors quand cette notion de personne peut être modifiée par la science ? Que deviennent des concepts aussi fondamentaux que la vie, la mort, la parenté?"

The arduous task of answering the above and other related questions has been taken on by an emerging interdisciplinary field with still fluid boundaries,[63] namely bioethics. Bioethics belongs to an equally new branch of ethical philosophy, applied ethics, with which in the view of many ethicists it overlaps in terms of content to such an extent,[64] that the two terms are sometimes used indistinguishably.[65] However, considering that bioethics is the result of very specific developments in the fields of medicine, biology, life sciences and biotechnology,[66] since "modern technology has introduced actions of such novel scale, objects, and consequences that the framework of former ethics can no longer contain them,"[67] while at the same time it "raises moral questions that are not simply difficult in the familiar sense but are of an altogether different kind,"[68] the view has prevailed in the relevant literature that bioethics should be regarded as a separate, completely distinct subfield of applied ethics, since it is better suited to the peculiarities

[63] Jessica Prata Miller, "Introduction to Special Cluster on Feminist Health-Care Ethics Consultation," *APA Newsletters* 5, no. 2 (2006): 2.

[64] See Warren Thomas Reich, "The Word 'Bioethics': Its Birth and the Legacies of those Who Shaped It," *Kennedy Institute of Ethics Journal* 4, no. 4 (1994): 319-335.

[65] See, for example, Peter Singer, *Practical Ethics* (Cambridge: Cambridge University Press, 1999), 344, 358, and Tristram Engelhardt Jr., *The Foundations of Bioethics* (Oxford: Oxford University Press, 1996), 9.

[66] See Dónal P. O'Mathúna, "Bioethics and Biotechnology," *Cytotechnology* 53, nos. 1-3 (2007): 113-119.

[67] Hans Jonas, *The Imperative of Responsibility: In Search of an Ethics for the Technological Age* (Chicago: University of Chicago Press, 1984), 6.

[68] Jürgen Habermas, *The Future of Human Nature* (Cambridge: Polity Press, 2003), 14. For the overwhelmingly extensive scope of bioethics and the challenges it poses, see Julian Savulescu, and Evangelos D. Protopapadakis, "Ethical Minefields and the Voice of Common Sense: A Discussion with Julian Savulescu," *Conatus – Journal of Philosophy* 4, no. 1 (2019): 125-133.

and requirements of this particular field. In what follows, I will not refer to bioethics as identical with applied ethics, but as one of its sub-fields.

a. A child of necessity

As is usual with the children of necessity, the circumstances surrounding the birth of bioethics were rather grim: The celebration of the end of World War II and the victory over evil was soon followed by the horror of what and how great that evil actually was. The images and film footage showing thousands of skeletal bodies stacked one on top of each other in the Nazi asylums and death camps, and the testimonies of the victims who were lucky enough to leave the camps alive, revealed the extent of the evil of which man is capable of. It also became clear that the atrocities and the crimes that were uncovered were, at least to a considerable extent, associated with scientists and doctors: Large-scale elimination of 'life unworthy of living,'[69] abuses in medical experiments on human subjects,[70] trials of experimental drugs, surgical procedures on inmates, monstrous studies of the limits of the human body,[71] forgery and falsification of death certificates and other official medical documents, you name it.[72] All of this was carried out

---

[69] See Erika Silvestri, "Lebensunwertes Leben: Roots and Memory of Aktion T4," *Conatus – Journal of Philosophy* 4, no. 2 (2019): 65-82.

[70] See Sheena M. Eagan, "Normalizing Evil: The National Socialist Physicians Leagues," *Conatus – Journal of Philosophy* 4, no. 2 (2019): 233-243.

[71] For a good discussion on the experiments on inmates, as well as on the justification of the experimentation, see Dimitra Chousou, Daniela Theodoridou, George Boutlas, Anna Batistatou, Christos Yapijakis, and Maria Syrrou, "Eugenics between Darwin's Era and the Holocaust," *Conatus – Journal of Philosophy* 4, no. 2 (2019): 171-204.

[72] For a detailed account see Tessa Chelouche, and Geoffrey Brahmer, *Casebook on Bioethics and the Holocaust* (Haifa: UNESCO Chair in

by physicians, biologists, geneticists, and in general by professionals who until then enjoyed the highest possible prestige, and to whom people's lives and health were entrusted, usually without reservation and without questioning their authority.[73] It became immediately clear that a paradigm shift was urgently needed in terms of the space given to scientists and physicians to decide and act for themselves, who should henceforth be bound by certain laws and regulations, and also be accountable to society. The *Nuremberg Code*, published in 1947, stemmed from the Nuremberg Tribunal and the so-called Doctors' Trials convened to judge the crimes against humanity committed by the Nazis during this period. The Code sought to establish the criteria that should be met in order for scientific experimentation on human subjects to be considered scientifically and ethically permissible; it was the first time that explicit reference was made to the voluntary consent of the human subjects:

> The voluntary consent of the human subject is absolutely essential. This means that the person involved should have legal capacity to give consent; should be so situated as to be able to exercise free power of choice, without the intervention of any element of force, fraud, deceit, duress, overreaching, or other ulterior form of constraint or

Bioethics, 2013); also, Stacy Gallin, and Ira Bedzow, eds., *Bioethics and the Holocaust: A Comprehensive Study in How the Holocaust Continues to Shape the Ethics of Health, Medicine and Human Rights* (Cham: Springer, 2022).

[73] For the role of physicians in the Holocaust see Mark A. Levine, Matthew K. Wynia, Meleah Himber, and William S. Silvers, "Pertinent Today: What Contemporary Lessons Should be Taught by Studying Physician Participation in the Holocaust?" *Conatus – Journal of Philosophy* 4, no. 2 (2019): 287-302.

coercion; and should have sufficient knowledge and comprehension of the elements of the subject matter involved as to enable him to make an understanding and enlightened decision.[74]

Together with the 1948 *United Nations Universal Declaration of Human Rights*, which recognizes the inherent dignity of all human beings, and understands their equal and inalienable rights as the foundation of freedom, justice and peace,[75] "the Nuremberg Code was to be the model shaping, to this day, the codes that aim to regulate biomedical experimentation on human subjects."[76] Another milestone in this process is, of course, the *Declaration of Helsinki* issued by the World Medical Association in 1967 – and since then revised and updated seven times. It places particular emphasis on autonomy, informed consent, and protection of the interests of the individual, especially in non-therapeutic clinical research.[77]

The key concepts that constitute the backbone of bioethics are already present in these documents; the coining of the term 'bioethics,' though, is usually dated to 1970-71 and attributed to Van Rensselaer Potter, although this is incorrect. The first mention of the term is found in a 1927 article by Fritz Jahr,[78] a Protestant theologian from Saxony, but with a com-

[74] Article one. "The Nuremberg Code," *British Medical Journal* 313 (1996): 1448.

[75] United Nations, *Universal Declaration of Human Rights*, https://www.un.org/en/about-us/universal-declaration-of-human-rights.

[76] A. F. Cascais, "Bioethics: History, Scope, Object," *Global Bioethics* 10, nos. 1-4 (1997): 11.

[77] World Medical Association, "Declaration of Helsinki: Ethical Principles for Medical Research Involving Human Subjects," *Bulletin of the World Health Organization* 79, no. 4 (2001): 373-374.

[78] Fernando Lolas, "Bioethics and Animal Research. A Personal Perspective and a Note on the Contribution of Fritz Jahr," *Biological Research* 41 (2008):

pletely different meaning than that used today.[79] Specifically, Jahr understood bioethics as the science that has the task of defining the human being's moral duties, not only toward her fellow humans, but also toward all living creatures and organisms, including animals and plants.[80] Although Jahr's understanding of bioethics has long been marginalized, it remains somewhat influential among bioethicists today, who refer to their approach as 'integrative bioethics.'[81]

Half a century later, in 1970, the term reappeared in the literature with an article by Van Rensselaer Potter, a biochemist and professor of oncology at the University of Wisconsin-Madison, entitled *Bioethics: Science of Survival*,[82] and a year later with his book *Bioethics: Bridge to the Future*.[83] In both his works Potter, just like Jahr before him, gave bioethics a much broader meaning than it

120.

[79] Hans-Martin Sass, "Fritz Jahr's 1927 Concept of Bioethics," *Kennedy Institute of Ethics Journal* 17, no. 4 (2007): 281.

[80] Fritz Jahr, "Bio-Ethik. Eine Umschau über die ethischen Beziehungen des Menschen zu Tier und Pflanze," *Kosmos: Handweiser für Naturfreunde* 24, no. 1 (1927): 2: "Under these circumstances it is only consequent when R. Eisler in summarizing uses the term Bio-Psychik (soul science of all life forms). It is only a small step from here to Bio-Ethics [Bio-Ethik, highlighted by Jahr], i.e., the assumption of moral duties not only towards humans but to all living beings as well," [translation by Sass, 281]; also, Florian Steger, "Fritz Jahr's (1895-1953) European concept of bioethics and its application potential," *Jahr* 6, no. 2 (2015): 217: "All life forms including animals and plants should be treated as ends in themselves as far as possible and not at all times, as demanded by Kant apropos of human beings."

[81] See Jos Schaefer-Rolffs, "Integrative Bioethics as a Chance: An Ideal Example for Ethical Discussions?" *Synthesis Philosophica* 53, no. 1 (2012): 107-122.

[82] Van Rensselaer Potter, "Bioethics, the Science of Survival," *Perspectives in Biology and Medicine* 14, no. 1 (1970): 127-153.

[83] Van Rensselaer Potter, *Bioethics: Bridge to the Future* (Englewood Cliffs, NJ: Prentice Hall, 1971).

has today. In particular, he understood bioethics as a science of survival in the ecological sense,[84] that is, as interdisciplinary research aimed at ensuring the existence and well-being of the biosphere.[85] Potter's conception of both the content of the concept and the goal of bioethics was never adopted, for otherwise the nascent discipline would obviously had led not only to overlaps with ecology but also with an extremely dynamic branch of applied ethics that had already become firmly established in the last quarter of the twentieth century, namely environmental ethics.[86]

As early as 1971, when Andre Hellegers founded the first institute for bioethics, the Joseph and Rose Kennedy Institute for the Study of Human Reproduction and Bioethics,[87] bioethics was turning more toward developments in medicine, genetics, and biotechnology. For Hellegers, bioethics should be the discipline that combines medical and ethical knowledge, and a mediator between the respective sciences.[88]

b. What it is

Since then and up to the present day, bioethics has received various definitions, in the context of which its subject matter is sometimes very closely related to that of medical ethics – either because bioethics is seen as an offshoot of the latter,[89] or because it is considered a completely related discipline.[90]

---

[84] Potter, "Bioethics, the Science of Survival," 136.

[85] Helga Kuhse, and Peter Singer, *A Companion to Bioethics* (New York: John Willey and Sons, 2009), 3.

[86] See Richard Routley, "Is There a Need for a New, an Environmental Ethic?" *Proceedings of the XVth World Congress of Philosophy* 1 (1973): 205-210.

[87] See Albert R. Jonsen, *The Birth of Bioethics* (New York: Oxford University Press, 2003), 22ff.

[88] Reich, 324.

[89] Kuhse, and Singer.

[90] *The Concise Routledge Encyclopedia of Philosophy*.

Sometimes, again, the boundaries of bioethics are extended to include ecological, environmental and economic issues related to the survival of our species,[91] apparently under the influence of the early concepts of bioethics by Jahr and Potter mentioned earlier. At other times the boundaries of bioethics are drawn more narrowly to include only issues of biomedicine and biotechnology.[92]

In any case, however, all approaches contribute to the following: [a] bioethics is an interdisciplinary field, and a meeting place for disciplines such as ethics, law, biology, medicine, genetics, biomedicine, and so on, [b] the primacy – due to the nature of the subject – belongs to ethics,[93] [c] the need to deal with bioethics arises from the rapid development in the field of the so-called *life sciences*,[94] [d] the subject of bioethics are the ethical problems arising from the developments in the field of these sciences, namely medicine, biology and genetic engineering, and the impact of these developments on human beings from an ethical point of view, religious, social, societal, political and legal aspects, [e] the aim of bioethics is to address these ethical problems in such a way that, on the one hand, the actual or potential risks of these developments to human

---

[91] Usually under the name "integrative bioethics." See, for example, Stephen O. Sodeke, and Wylin D. Wilson, "Integrative Bioethics is a Bridge-Builder Worth Considering to Get Desired Results," *American Journal of Bioethics* 17, no. 9 (2017): 30-32; also Schaefer-Rolffs.

[92] Peter Kemp, and Jacob Dahl Rendtorff, "The Barcelona Declaration," *Synthesis Philosophica* 46, no. 2 (2008): 245: "[...] ethical questions raised by the progress in modern biomedicine and biotechnology."

[93] Richard Huxtable, "Friends, Foes, Flatmates: On the Relationship between Law and Bioethics," in *Empirical Bioethics: Practical and Theoretical Perspectives*, eds. J. Ives, M. Dunn, and A. Cribb, 84-102 (Cambridge: Cambridge University Press, 2017), 87: "In short, bioethics is ethics, which is moral philosophy, albeit visiting the realm of the biosciences."

[94] *The Concise Routledge Encyclopedia of Philosophy*.

dignity, health, and well-being are limited and, on the other hand, the acquisition of new knowledge and its beneficial application for the benefit of human beings are not impeded.

In short, bioethics can be defined as an interdisciplinary branch of applied ethics that examines and attempts to address old and new ethical issues that are either emerging, exacerbated, or reinterpreted by rapid developments in the life sciences (biology, genetics, medicine, biomedicine, biotechnology, and others) in order to achieve the best possible balance between scientific progress and the preservation of human values and well-being in the interest of humanity.

Moreover, it should be noted that the role of bioethics is not limited to merely theoretical discussions. The role of bioethics – through various committees, commissions, and other working bodies around the world – is usually also to find functional solutions to urgent and controversial practical issues that confront researchers and medical personnel in their daily practice. Bioethicists not infrequently find themselves in the uncomfortable position of having to make short-term decisions about serious issues that require immediate resolution. In most cases, the decisions made by these bodies are translated into state laws or deontological codes that govern the duties and responsibilities of professionals in biomedical research and practice. Because the dilemmas that bioethics must confront are sometimes extremely delicate and at the same time unprecedented, both legislative bodies and the public cannot avoid relying almost exclusively on the opinions of bioethicists.[95] Against this backdrop, bioethics often takes on much more institutional roles. This

---

[95] The power entrusted to bioethicists is sometimes discussed as 'bi-power;' see, among others, Lydia Tsiakiri, "Euthanasia: Promoter of Autonomy or Supporter of Biopower?" *Conatus – Journal of Philosophy* 7, no. 1 (2022): 123-133.

means that bioethicists generally do not have the luxury of exploring exotic views, as ethicists in other fields do; instead, they must be much more careful about the conclusions they reach and the suggestions they make. This also means that bioethics needs general guidelines, norms that provide at least some directions and exclude others.

c. Norms and principles

Ethics can either be agent-oriented, focusing on the character traits of the moral agent that indicate virtues or vices, or action-oriented, focusing on whether particular actions are consistent with moral duties or entail the best possible consequences. By its very nature, bioethics seems to be indifferent to virtues and vices. Its only concern is whether this or that application of a particular biotechnological advance is compatible with what we consider ethically significant, especially with our moral understanding of duties, rights, and values, or the extent to which it promotes what we consider to be the common good. And while agent-oriented ethics allows for some flexibility in moral evaluation, action-oriented ethics depends to a considerable extent on norms and principles. Given the special nature of the field, the various demands that arise from it, and its institutional importance, it has been felt that it would be useful, if not necessary, for bioethics to agree on a rough outline of certain general principles that should govern bioethics.

The so-called *Belmont Report*[96] of September 30, 1978,

---

[96] The actual title of the report is: *Ethical Principles and Guidelines for the Protection of Human Subjects of Research, Report of the National Commission for the Protection of Human Subjects of Biomedical and Behavioral Research*; see https://www.hhs.gov/ohrp/regulations-and-policy/belmont-report/read-the-belmont-report/index.html.

was the first attempt to establish general guidelines for the rapidly evolving field of biomedical research, thereby providing a safety net for those who might be affected, particularly patients and people who participate as subjects in biomedical research. Commission members agreed on three basic ethical principles: [1] respect for personal autonomy (especially by ensuring informed consent of those involved in biomedical research), [2] beneficence (minimizing risks and maximizing benefits), and [3] justice (fair and equal distribution of costs and benefits).

A year later, in 1979, Tom Beauchamp and James Childress published the first edition of their *Principles of Biomedical Ethics* – now in its 7th edition,[97] which popularized *principlism* as a response to the ethical issues arising from biomedical research and practice. In their work, Beauchamp and Childress propose a four principles approach to biomedical ethics, one that they believe can be helpful by providing guidelines for ethical decision-making about dilemmas that arise in the field. These principles are: [1] respect for autonomy (a norm of respecting the decision-making capacities of autonomous persons),[98] [2] beneficence (a group of norms for providing benefits and balancing benefits against risks and costs),[99] [3] non-maleficence (a norm of avoiding the causation of harm),[100] and [4] justice (a group of norms for distributing benefits, risks and costs fairly).[101] These have been proposed as abstract moral norms that could provide action-guiding content, and it is argued that they are

---

[97] Tom L. Beauchamp, and James Childress, *Principles of Biomedical Ethics* (New York: Oxford University Press, 2012).

[98] Ibid., 38.

[99] Ibid.

[100] Ibid.

[101] Ibid.

compatible with a wide variety of moral theories
that are often themselves mutually incompatible.
[…] a way forward in the context of intercultural
ethics, that treads the delicate path between moral relativism and moral imperialism,[102]

because "in another framework they might be developed as
'rights,' 'virtues,' or 'values.'"[103] The issue of compatibility is obviously of enormous importance, since one of the main goals
of bioethics is to achieve the broadest possible acceptance and
applicability,[104] therefore Beauchamp and Childress spare no
effort to demonstrate that each of the four principles they propose could be endorsed by a wide range of ethicists regardless
of whether they are under the influence of completely different
ethical traditions. The most telling example of this is their discussion of respect for autonomy, a principle that, in their view,
can be accepted by otherwise completely diverse ethical views,
such as the moral theories of Kant and Mill.[105]

The principles suggested by Beauchamp and Childress, in
elaborated form, serve as the backbone for the final text of the
Universal Declaration on Bioethics and Human Rights adopted
at the General Conference of UNESCO on October 12, 2005,
which states: [1] respect for human dignity and human rights
– together with respect for fundamental human freedoms –

---

[102] Raanan Gillon, "Ethics Needs Principles – Four Can Encompass the Rest
– and Respect for Autonomy Should Be 'First among Equals,'" *Journal of
Medical Ethics* 29 (2003): 307.

[103] Beauchamp, and Childress, 37.

[104] Raanan Gillon, "The Four Principles Revisited – A Reappraisal," in
Principles of Health Care Ethics, ed. R. Gillon, 319-333 (London: John Wiley,
1994), 326.

[105] Beauchamp, and Childress, 125.

must be absolute, on the one hand, and must take precedence over the interests of society, on the other; [2] bioethics must be characterized by the principle of beneficence, viz. maximizing the benefits and minimizing the harms from the application and advancement of scientific knowledge, medical practices, and related technologies for the benefit of patients, those involved in scientific research, and those affected by it; [3] it must also be guided by the principle of autonomy and individual responsibility in decision making, and the protection of the rights and interests of persons who are unable to exercise them should be paramount; [4] free and informed consent should be required for preventive, diagnostic, and therapeutic medical interventions, as well as in the context of scientific research, and it should be possible to revoke consent without consequences for the person revoking it; [5] special care should be taken to protect individuals who are unable to give consent for various reasons, in the interest of their health and in accordance with the protection of the human rights of the individual; [6] respect for the vulnerability of individuals and their personal integrity, on the basis of which vulnerable individuals and groups should be protected; [7] privacy and confidentiality of personal data must be respected; [8] equality, equity and fairness must be upheld; [9] the avoidance of discrimination and stigmatization of individuals or groups on any grounds must be promoted, while non-violation of human dignity and human rights must be ensured; [10] respect for multiculturalism and pluralism must be promoted, provided that such respect does not constitute a violation of human rights and does not conflict with other principles of the Declaration; [11] efforts must be made to promote solidarity among peoples and to consolidate international cooperation; [12] social responsibility must be promoted, and health protected; [13] the participation of the

entire international community in the benefits arising from
scientific research and its applications must be ensured; [14]
future generations, in particular their genetic heritage, must be
protected; and [15] the environment, the biosphere, and biological diversity must be protected.[106]

d. Not just ethics

In the case of bioethics, however, norms and principles cannot simply be conceived as ethical concepts in a vacuum. Rapid advances in science and technology over the past century
have exacerbated existing ethical problems, sometimes giving
them a new form, and making them even more complex and
difficult to resolve. Intellectual property theft and pedophilia,
for example, have always been the subject of moral and legal
concerns. However, with the widespread use of the Internet,
they have taken on a new dynamic and new aspects, as both
can now be done much more easily and effectively. Euthanasia, on the other hand, was already mentioned as a practice as
early as in the Hippocratic Oath. Nowadays, however, it has
emerged with a new dynamic. This is because the possibilities
of modern medicine and the development of medical technology now allow doctors to keep a patient in a vegetative state
alive for as long as they see fit, which was not possible just
a few years ago.[107] However, this does not make euthanasia a
new moral issue.

However, in addition to long-standing concerns, certain
developments in biomedicine, biotechnology, and genetics

---

[106] UNESCO, *Universal Declaration on Bioethics and Human Rights* (Paris:
UNESCO, 2006), 5-7.
[107] For an insightful discussion see Jose Luis Guerrero Quiñones, "Physicians'
Role in Helping to Die," *Conatus – Journal of Philosophy* 7, no. 1 (2022): 79-
101.

have created new ethical dilemmas. Societies usually become aware of these dilemmas only after the scientific advances that produce them have already been completed, and therefore take everybody by surprise. They often become points of intense scientific and social conflict, are emotionally charged, and plunge us into a state of confusion as they challenge entrenched concepts and attitudes.[108] Today, it is technologically possible to create clones, exact copies of existing organisms – both animal and human – through nuclear transfer and genetic manipulation of somatic cells, which was impossible in the past. Geneticists today also claim that they can alter the human genome to achieve not only very specific phenotypic traits, but also to influence the character and behavior of the individual. Today, it is also possible for a woman to carry a child to whom she has no genetic connection or relationship. At the same time, she could simply have such a child without even carrying it to term, since the task of gestation can now be entrusted to a surrogate mother. These and similar considerations present new moral questions that are *terra incognita* for moral thought. These considerations are accompanied by the expected questions that arise in and around any scientific achievement if it is to be put into practice, and which always boil down to the question of whether the achievement under consideration should pass from the stage of scientific possibility to that of *in rem* application, to what extent this must be the case, what guarantees must accompany the application of scientific knowledge, how far this application may go, and so on.

In other words, bioethics today, even when it addresses novel ethical dilemmas such as cloning, can only examine

---

[108] Indicative of the – sometimes – unwarranted tensions that accompany questions of bioethics is Singer's description of the protests by activists in Germany when he was invited to give a lecture at the University of Hamburg. See Singer, *Practical Ethics*, 338-339.

them in terms of asking traditional questions. And this is quite reasonable, for bioethics is at its core and essence a branch of ethics, and ethics cannot avoid asking primarily practical questions – or at least questions that relate to practical problems. Ethical views and theories also have a peculiarity that makes their justification quite demanding: They are judged not only at the level of their theoretical coherence and validity, but also at the level of their practical application – unlike other branches of philosophy, such as metaphysics, where the test to which any approach is subjected can only be theoretical.

If bioethics hopes to provide satisfactory answers to traditional or new ethical problems, it must adopt practices that are unusual to traditional, theoretical ethics. It must work closely with and be informed by the relevant sciences for two reasons. First, progress in the sciences has changed – and continues to change – the content of basic concepts that were once taken for granted: For example, it is not entirely clear today what is meant by the terms 'mother,' 'father,' 'death,' 'life,' and others. Is a patient who is kept in a vegetative state only by mechanical means alive or not? She is certainly not dead, at least not as dead as a corpse. On the other hand, she is not alive either, at least not as you or I are. So is she a human being – especially a moral person?[109] If not, then why do we, in most cases, believe that we have certain moral obligations to her, and also assume that she remains the bearer of some moral rights?[110] Is the woman who carries an embryo resulting from the in vitro treatment of a somatic cell whose nucleus has been removed and inserted into the ovum of another woman, unknown to

---

[109] Quoted in Stanley I. Benn, "Abortion, Infanticide and Respect for Persons," in *The Problem of Abortion*, ed. Joel Feinberg, 92-104 (Belmont, CA: Wadsworth Publishing Company, 1973), 99-100.

[110] Kirsten Rabe Smolensky, "The Rights of the Dead," *Hofstra Law Review* 37 (2009): 764.

her, and implanted in her uterus, the mother of the embryo she carries?[111] Does the alteration of the genome, which produces not only a desired phenotype but a genetic predisposition to the occurrence of certain behaviors, constitute a *legitimate intervention* in one's personality on a par with previously accepted practices such as positive eugenics[112] and intensive and targeted education,[113] or is it an intervention of a different kind that directly affects what we call, perhaps vaguely, *value* or *dignity* of the human being? Does genetic programming create a different type of human being with limited options for action and decision-making that is fixed into a predetermined future,[114] and thus violates the right to an *open future* as understood by many?[115] Any satisfactory treatment of such questions requires the help of philosophy, medicine, biology, psychology, ethics, law, etc.

Second, if bioethics is not adequately informed by the sciences, it runs the risk of reducing its potential to bland discussions that not only have no utility in solving the ethical problem at hand, but rather confuse and disorient. As a typical example, I would cite the debate over cloning dictators, criminals, or docile armies of serial killers. This debate has been going on for a long time – and to some extent continues to-

---

[111] See, inter alia, Randall P. Bezanson, "Solomon Would Weep: A Comment on In the Matter of Baby M and the Limits of Judicial Authority," *The Journal of Law, Medicine & Ethics* 16, nos. 1-2 (1988): 126-130.

[112] David McCarthy, "Persons and Their Copies," *Journal of Medical Ethics* 25 (1999): 99.

[113] See Habermas, especially 49ff.

[114] Allen Buchanan, Daniel Brock, Norman Daniels, and Daniel Winkler, *From Chance to Choice: Genetics and Justice* (Cambridge: Cambridge University Press, 2001), 178.

[115] See Joel Feinberg, "The Child's Right to an Open Future," in *Who's Child? Children's Rights, Parental Authority and State Power*, eds. William Aiken, and Hugh LaFollete, 124-153 (Totowa, NJ: Littlefield, Adams and Co., 1980).

day – despite the relevant findings of genetics and psychology, which lead to the following conclusions: [a] the possibilities of cloning are limited to the production of identical phenotypes, but in no case can human cloning produce mental duplicates, as the case of identical twins clearly shows: Although they have identical genetic material and develop in the same family, social and natural environment, they never seem to have identical character traits,[116] and [b] genotype is only one of the parameters that determine one's personality, in the formation of which the social and historical environment, upbringing and also luck play an equally important – if not more important – role, and therefore, no matter how many times, for example, Adolf Hitler or Idi Amin Dada were cloned, not a single one of them would result in the same bloodthirsty tyrant.[117] As Neil Levy and Miana Lotz aptly note, the genome does not play as important a role in shaping personality as we

---

[116] Bernard E. Rollin, "Keeping up with the Cloneses: Issues in Human Cloning," *The Journal of Ethics* 3, no. 1 (1999): 62: "[…] as if cloning were a form of xeroxing all aspects of a human being's physical, mental, personality, and social traits. This is, of course, a highly misleading analogy. First of all, we have the evidence of natural clones – 'identical' twins. Not only do identical twins have the same genetic structure, they are often raised in as close to the same environment as humans can be raised. Yet, though they may end up similar in many ways, they also end up dissimilar, in indefinite numbers of other ways. Certainly, they are not the same person, thinking the same thoughts at the same moment."

[117] See, for example, John Harris, "*Goodbye Dolly?* The Ethics of Human Cloning," *Journal of Medical Ethics* 23, no. 6 (1997): 357ff: "[...] Moreover, the futility of any such attempt is obvious. Hitler's genotype might conceivably produce a 'gonadically challenged' individual of limited stature, but reliability in producing an evil and vicious megalomaniac is far more problematic," and Habermas, 124, n. 54: "[...] manipulation has been carried out with the sole intention of acting on the phenotypic molding of a specific genetic program, and this of course on condition that the technologies required for this goal have proved to be successful."

sometimes think: After all, no gene responsible for conservatism or Catholicism has yet been identified.[118] So not only has the debate been conducted in a way that has rendered it irrelevant and thus useless, but it has also, in my opinion, distracted us from other, more concrete ethical issues about cloning.[119]

Despite all that I have said about the importance and role of other sciences for the adequacy and effectiveness of bioethics, it should not escape us that the dominant role in this discipline belongs to ethics, which is the core of bioethics. For, in my opinion, while the role of the sciences is of paramount importance, namely to nourish and keep ethical thinking up to date, any decision about the ethical dilemmas that bioethics seeks to answer can only be ethical in the first place: Bioethical decisions are about gains and losses, imminent risks and promising prospects, balancing the interests of the whole against those of the individual – whenever and wherever these come into conflict. Above all, bioethics has the task of drawing boundaries, of showing us how far we should venture – and how deep – in the brave new world that science and technology promise us. Any question that involves an 'ought' can only be an ethical question. Against this background, in the following I will deal with one of the most heated current bioethical debates, namely the one about human reproductive cloning,

---

[118] Neil Levy, and Miana Lotz, "Reproductive Cloning and a (Kind of) Genetic Fallacy," *Bioethics* 19, no. 3 (2005): 237ff. See also Jaime Ahlberg, and Harry Brighouse, "An Argument Against Cloning," *Canadian Journal of Philosophy* 40, no. 4 (2010): 541ff.

[119] Rollin, 53: "The lesson here is simple. In the absence of good, reflective, careful ethical thinking about technology initiated by those who introduce a technology, and who should (in principle) understand it well enough to think through its implications, the social-ethical lacuna created by the technology will be filled by sensationalistic, simplistic, emotionally-based slogans which dominate social thought and whose intuitive appeal make them difficult to dislodge."

and discuss it from an ethical point of view – but by no means neglecting the relevant data that the sciences provide.

III. Uniqueness and dignity

Let me start with this: There are no unique copies. Once something is a copy, it can only be the copy of something else, so it cannot be unique – and vice versa: Anything that is unique cannot be the copy – that is, an exact replication – of something else. The title of this book may therefore strike one as a blatant and glaring contradiction – or better yet, as an oxymoron: Either the clone of an existing being is unique and thus not a clone, or it is a copy and thus not unique; *tertium non datur*. So, the question can be either: Are we able to create unique beings? or: Are we able to create exact copies? And while the answer to the first question is clear, the answer to the second question is much more doubtful and controversial.

The task of providing answers to the above questions clearly lies with scientists, not ethicists; the only question to which ethics really needs to provide an answer can only be: Why should concerns about uniqueness be morally relevant when it comes to cloning? Indeed, the question of uniqueness seems to acquire its unparalleled moral significance only when the focus of the debate is limited to human replication – it would be a platitude to claim that ingrained in us is the tendency (some would say *bias*) to assume that our own uniqueness is something *unique*, which makes anything that might compromise or nullify that uniqueness at least morally questionable. Although this view has been strongly challenged by ethicists and scientists alike, especially in the last century, it still prevails. Nevertheless, the notion that humans are unique in a way that living beings of other species are not raises several questions.

First, the view that humans are unique does not mean that the species homo sapiens is unique among all other species; after all, *every species* is unique in this respect. Rather, it means that each and every human being is *fundamentally* different and distinct from each and every other human being – as opposed to, say, individual horses or chipmunks, which are not fundamentally different or distinct from other horses or chipmunks. Again, this view seems to be supported neither by common experience, nor by reason. On the one hand, our senses and our science tell us that every individual being, regardless of the species to which it belongs, is different and distinct from every other of its kind – in this sense, every single horse is also unique, no less than any human: larger or smaller, more or less intelligent, faster or slower, even slightly genetically different from any other, and so on. On the other hand, reason tells us that if two things are numerically different, then there must be at least one property that is not shared by both – this is the point of McTaggart's law of *dissimilarity of the diverse*: If two things are diverse, then there must be at least one property that one has and the other does not.[120] This applies equally to humans, horses and chipmunks, but also to blades of grass, as Leibnitz illustrates this view.[121] It follows

---

[120] John McTaggart Ellis McTaggart, *The Nature of Existence* (Cambridge: Cambridge University Press, 1988), vol. 1, §94. The law (or principle) of the *Dissimilarity of the Diverse* is McTaggart's explanation of the law of the *Identity of Indiscernibles* by Leibniz. For an excellent account – and refutation – see C. D. Broad, "McTaggart's Principle of the Dissimilarity of the Diverse," *Proceedings of the Aristotelian Society*, 1931 - 1932, New Series 32 (1931 – 1932): 41-52.

[121] For a good discussion on Leibniz's law of the identity of the indiscernibles see Ari Maunu, "Indiscernibility of Identicals and Substitutivity in Leibniz," *History of Philosophy Quarterly* 19, no. 4 (2002): 367-380. For more on the implications of Leibniz's law in regard to human reproductive cloning see chapter ….

that the view that humans are unique in a way that other creatures are not – the core of our much revered uniqueness that
makes human reproductive cloning morally unacceptable, but
not cattle or plant cloning – should be based on some *further
fact*, but certainly not on empirical facts or logical conclusions. The question remains: Are there reasons that justify the
claim that the uniqueness of human beings is of *such a special
nature* that it deserves special moral treatment?

Since quantitative and/or qualitative uniqueness applies
equally to all beings and things anyway, what do we mean
when we say that humans are unique, unless we are slipping
into a cliché? There must be at least one quality that makes
each of us unique in a special way, but that cannot be *our particular uniqueness*: In this respect, we can only be identical
– the notion of human uniqueness is, after all, based on the
assumption that it is a trait that all members of our species
share simply because of their human nature. At this point, it
would be useful to discuss in more detail what we mean by
uniqueness, because it seems that most arguments against human reproductive cloning that focus on potential implications
for human uniqueness betray a kind of conceptual confusion
about this concept, uniqueness.

a. Uniqueness as distinctiveness vs. uniqueness as superiority

When we postulate that this or that being or thing is unique,
we may mean that it is something of which *there is only one*, the
only one of its kind that has either ever existed, or the only one
that time has preserved for us to contemplate in the present. In
this sense Michelangelo Buonarroti's statue of David is unique
because Michelangelo never created another sculpture of David. In the second sense, the only intact skull of one of our ancestors, the Neanderthal, would be unique, because it is the only

one of numerous others to have survived the malice of time. But that is not the only meaning of the term *unique*.

Unique can also mean that something, while it is not that of which there is only one, yet it *stands alone* compared to others of its kind because of its unparalleled excellence in some quality. In this sense, the statue of David would again be unique, not because there are no other statues of David by sculptors other than Michelangelo, but because we consider *this* statue to be by far the most outstanding because of its superior excellence in one aspect – or in all aspects. The Neanderthal skull, in turn, would again be unique not because it is the only skull we have, but because it is the only *intact* skull, and this quality of it, at least from the point of view of anthropologists, is synonymous with it being outstanding.[122]

In both respects, anything that is unique is also *unparalleled* and, therefore, *precious*: If that of which there is only one is lost or destroyed, an entire *ontological* category is lost and destroyed; and if that which stands alone in comparison to others of its kind is lost and destroyed, an entire *aesthetic* category is lost and destroyed. The difference is that what we reveal when we use the term in the descriptive sense is merely *a pragmatic judgement* by which we declare a basic fact, to wit that there is *no other of this kind*, whereas in the other sense we ascribe some kind of praise to what we classify as unique, that is, that there is *no better of this kind*.[123] In other words, any premise that states that something is unique, can be either descriptive, i.e., a statement about what is, or prescriptive or normative, i.e., a statement about how it should be contemplated, understood, or treated.

---

[122] See "unique, adj. and n.," *Oxford English Dictionary Online*. Oxford University Press, March 2015, http://www.oed.com/view/Entry/214712.

[123] Davidson, "Human Uniqueness," 218.

When it comes to the uniqueness of human beings, I think the phrases 'every human being is unique' or 'human beings are unique' are used in both these meanings simultaneously: On the one hand, the term describes the fact that every human being is genetically, phenotypically, and also with regard to its character distinct to any other human being who has ever existed, currently exists, or will exist in the future, and on the other hand, as Davidson puts it, that "human beings belong in a different, superior, and indeed incomparable, order from the rest of creation."[124] The attribution of this quality, uniqueness, to human beings could at the same time be taken as *both* descriptive and prescriptive: On the one hand it reveals an empirical truth about the members of the species *Homo sapiens*, and at the same time it tells us how we should think about them and treat them.

The whole discussion so far boils down to the fact that being unique is being *unparalleled* either as standing out against all other beings of one's kind, or being the member of a 'superior, incomparable order'. The former is a good springboard for considering uniqueness as a reason for ascribing infinite value, as well as irreplaceability to any being that falls into this category; the latter is a reason for treating it with the highest possible moral respect – it doesn't take much to see that the latter is also to a large extend dependent upon the former. What it is it, then, that makes human beings unique, i.e., infinitely valuable, irreplaceable, and worthy of the highest possible moral respect, that is, distinctive and superior, in a sense that other beings are not? This question is of paramount importance here, for if cloning can compromise the uniqueness of the human being, then it should also be able to eliminate or

---

[124] Andrew Davison, "Human Uniqueness: Standing Alone?" *The Expository Times* 127, no. 5 (2016): 218.

nullify that which makes the human being one of the three, or all three at the same time.

It is true that all beings, regardless of the species to which they belong, are numerically distinct and at the same time substantially so, that is, quantitatively or qualitatively different from every other being of their kind. Humans are no different from rocks or starfish in this respect: Nowhere in nature are there two rocks or starfish that are identical in shape, chemical composition, color, and so on. However, although each rock and each starfish are unique in this sense, rocks and starfish are not generally considered to be infinitely valuable, irreplaceable, and worthy of the highest possible moral respect. With the exception of rocks that are hand-crafted by humans, rocks are not *valued* and are not *valuable*. Humans, on the other hand, are. This means that human beings are considered unique not as *instances of nature*, but because of something else perceived as interwoven with their very existence as the beings they are. Probably the most common explanation for this is that humans, unlike (most or even all) other beings, are *persons*, which is enough to make them unique in a sense that no other being can ever be.

b. Uniqueness and personhood

In view of the above, it is not humanity that makes each human unique, but *personhood* instead; given, though, that in the view of many *only* humans can be persons, humans are unique by virtue of their personhood.[125] Maybe because it

---

[125] "But 'person' signifies something singular [...]. Therefore also the *individuals* of the rational nature have a special name even among other substances; and this name is 'person.'" Thomas Aquinas, *Summa Theologica* (Notre Dame, IN: Christian Classics, 1981), Question 29, Article 1, Objection 1, and corpus.

sounds plausible, or because it is just convenient[126] to hold the view that humans, apart from being merely individual instances of nature, are also unique as *persons*, philosophers so far have rarely considered the implications of this view, and the questions that inevitably come together with it. Nevertheless, this view gives rise to a series of pressing questions that need to be answered before it is accepted as a good basis for establishing human uniqueness. Firstly, are *all* human beings persons and, hence, unique? Or some are not? Secondly, are *only* human beings persons, or might there be other beings, living or not, that could also be acknowledged the property of personhood, and hence be equally unique as humans are? Thirdly, and most importantly, what are the qualities any being must have to be entitled to personhood? As to the first and the second question, it is true that the fact that

> "Person" is not a term in the classification of nature […] makes it possible for philosophers like Michael Tooley and Peter Singer to deny that human fetuses and infants are persons, and for philosophers like Thomas White to attribute personhood to some animals […]. Of course, it could turn out that all and only humans are persons, but it takes an argument to defend that. Someone who claims that there are humans who are not persons or persons who are not human is not making a conceptual mistake.[127]

---

[126] As Peter Singer aptly notes, "Fellow-humans are unlikely to reject the accolades we so generously bestow on them, and those to whom we deny the honor are unable to object." Peter Singer, "All Animals Are Equal," in *Animal Ethics: Past and Present Perspectives*, ed. Evangelos D. Protopapadakis, 163-178 (Berlin: Logos Verlag, 2012), 173.

[127] Linda Zagzebski, "The Dignity of Persons and the Value of Uniqueness,"

As if the puzzle were not already difficult enough to solve, recent advances in the field of artificial intelligence are also prompting philosophers to explore the possibility of granting some sort of personhood to powerful algorithms that "take on cognitive work [...] previously performed by humans,"[128] or to a general artificial intelligence that might adapt itself so as to be 'significantly more generally applicable,' and thus be capable of evolving by reprograming itself according to the knowledge it would acquire through interaction with its environment. I think it almost goes without saying that before giving a convincing answer to these two questions, one should address the third, namely what it is that makes each being a person and, in this line of thought, unique. The traditional answers to the question: "What is it that distinguishes persons from non-persons in ontologically and morally significant ways?" usually focus on rationality, self-consciousness, agency, and incommunicability.[129]

i. Rationality

The emphasis on rationality was introduced by Boethius and soon became dominant in Western philosophy. According to the well-known definition proposed by Boethius, a person is

Proceedings and Addresses of the American Philosophical Association 90 (2016): 60.

[128] Nick Bostrom, and Eliezer Yudkowsky, "The Ethics of Artificial Intelligence," in The *Cambridge Handbook of Artificial Intelligence*, eds. Keith Frankish, and William M. Ramsey, 316-334 (Cambridge: Cambridge University Press, 2014), 317.

[129] For the latter, see Linda Zagzebski, "The Uniqueness of Persons," *Journal of Religious Ethics* 29, no. 3 (2001): 401-423, especially 414ff.

"naturae rationabilis individua substantia,"[130] that is, an individual substance of rational nature. Philosophers and scholars from Thomas Aquinas[131] to Immanuel Kant adopted the capacity for rationality as the key element of personhood. To Aquinas the term *person* "signifies what is most perfect in all nature – that is, a subsistent individual of a rational nature."[132] One should note here that both Boethius and Aquinas emphasize individuality as much as rationality; as I will show later, this also has a certain bearing upon our subject matter, human reproductive cloning. But to return to Aquinas' definition, the key notion here – that which is 'most perfect in all nature' – is rationality, since numerous other beings are 'subsistent individuals,' but not of 'rational nature.' This line of reasoning culminates in Kant's view on the interdependence of humanity, personhood, and rationality:

> Kant does not distinguish rationality from human nature, nor does he distinguish between one's humanity and one's personhood [...]. Kant confines dignity to human beings because, he says, human beings are the only creatures who carry the moral law within themselves. So it appears that Kant does not distinguish a person from an instance of rational nature; indeed, he does not distinguish a person from an instance of human nature.[133]

---

[130] Boethius, "Treatise against Eutyches and Nestorius," in *The Theological Tractates*, trans. H. F. Stewart, and E. K. Randch (London: W. Heinemann, 1918), chapter 3 (PL 64, col. 1343).

[131] Aquinas, Part I, Question 29, Article 1, Objection 1.

[132] Aquinas, Part I, Question 29, Article 3.

[133] Zagzebski, "The Dignity of Persons and the Value of Uniqueness," 62-63.

The attribution of personhood on the basis of rationality, however, still leaves us with several unanswered questions: In case humans *are not* the only rational beings, shouldn't we regard other non-human rational animals as persons, too, and hence unique in the sense we assume that humans are? Whales, dolphins, chimpanzees, pigs, and probably also dogs, some bird species, and several others make themselves excellent candidates to be included in this category. On the other hand, several human beings should also be denied the faculty of personhood on the same ground, since they obviously lack rationality: Infants, to start with, have not yet developed rationality, and embryos also, while elderly people with dementia, or intellectually handicapped humans, have been deprived of rationality due to their condition. Rationality seems to be no safe ground for establishing personhood; it provides space for denying the property of personhood to beings we are accustomed to think of as persons and forces us to acknowledge this quality to beings we seem reluctant to do so. But we might just be wrong in our moral intuitions concerning who should be considered a person, and who shouldn't. The real issue here is that rationality is being proposed as the sole criterion for personhood, but without being supported with good reasons: No good reason is provided about why it is rationality that should be considered as the basis of personhood, and not some other property. As a matter of fact, there cannot be any concrete justification why perfectly self-aware, sentient beings, although they are absolutely incapable of mastering logic, or elevating themselves above their impulses and instincts of their nature so as to harmonize their decisions and actions to any categorical imperative or moral law, shouldn't also be acknowledged personhood, at least to some extent.

ii. Self-consciousness

Self-consciousness would probably be a much more convenient answer to this, since it seems capable of including many beings that, although they are not rational – or, rational to the extent human beings are, nevertheless stand out as unique individuals against others of their kind as having self-reflective consciousness, that is, consciousness of themselves being conscious. According to John Locke the notion of personhood is to be distinguished from that of belonging to the human species:

> This being premised, to find wherein personal identity consists, we must consider what person stands for; which, I think, is a thinking intelligent being, that has reason and reflection, and can consider itself as itself, the same thinking thing, in different times and places; which it does only by that consciousness which is inseparable from thinking, and, as it seems to me, essential to it: it being impossible for anyone to perceive without perceiving that he does perceive. When we see, hear, smell, taste, feel, meditate, or will anything, we know that we do so. Thus it is always as to our present sensations and perceptions: and by this everyone is to himself that which he calls self – it not being considered, in this case, whether the same self be continued in the same or divers substances. For, since consciousness always accompanies thinking, and it is that which makes everyone to be what he calls self, and thereby distinguishes himself from all other thinking things, in this alone consists personal identity,

i.e., the sameness of a rational being: and as far as this consciousness can be extended backwards to any past action or thought, so far reaches the identity of that person; it is the same self now it was then; and it is by the same self with this present one that now reflects on it, that that action was done.[134]

It is clear that for Locke personhood is intimately connected with rationality, self-reflective consciousness, and memory – the latter being the fabric that enables the continuity of identity over time. As Zagzebski aptly notes, "Locke's proposal is an improvement over the Boethian definition, because it comes closer to capturing the important idea that a person is a 'who,' not a 'what.'"[135] Being an individual entity that regards itself as an 'I' that persists over time, however, does not say much about what that 'I' may be. Self-reflective consciousness may enable one to grasp one's self as an 'I' that persists over time, but identity (or personhood) is definitely not identical with the ability to grasp oneself as a continuous existence; the conception of personhood involves much more than self-reflective consciousness: When I say that *I* am the person I am, I mean not only that I am able to conceive of myself as a continuous existence across time, but rather that I have certain likes and dislikes, inclinations, talents, that I perceive the world in a certain, unique way, that I occupy a certain space that no one else could occupy at the same time and, hence, my viewpoint is absolutely unique, that I have established certain relationships with my environment and other beings, and so on. Zag-

---

[134] John Locke, *An Essay Concerning Human Understanding*, ed. Roger Woolhouse (London: Penguin, 1997), II, xxvii, 9.

[135] Zagzebski, "The Uniqueness of Persons," 407.

zebski argues that Aristotle's *Unmoved Mover* also has self-reflective consciousness, this being probably its only feature;[136] but would this suffice for it to count as a person? Zagzebski thinks not, and I am inclined to think the same. Self-awareness is probably together with memory among the most essential components of personhood, but they are by no means *identical* with it. This view might also be supported by the fact that moral intuition usually favors ascribing the quality of personhood to human beings who have either not yet developed self-consciousness, or have long been deprived of it, such as embryos and infants on the one hand, and patients in an irreversible coma on the other. That being said, most people are also often not at all averse to granting self-consciousness to animals such as dogs, cats, chimpanzees and dolphins, even though they might not be equally willing to grant them full personhood, at least not in the sense that human beings are granted it. In short, self-consciousness may be a prerequisite for being classified as a person, but it cannot be the only criterion.

iii. Agency

Another traditional approach to the question of the grounds on which personhood – and thus, uniqueness – can be ascribed to any being, focuses on the capacity for agency, the capacity to act *for* and *towards* ends that have been set by the agent herself, and are not determined externally or by one's own nature. In this respect humans, unlike all other living beings, have the capacity "to act on the basis of self-imposed principles and therefore [...] in the logical space of practical reasons."[137] In short, while

---

[136] Ibid., see 406, 408.

[137] Henry Allison, *Kant's Groundwork for the Metaphysics of Morals: A Commentary* (Oxford: Oxford University Press, 2011), 308.

creatures other than human can only *react* to stimuli – either internal or external, such as inclinations, instincts, desires, or challenges posed by the environment, humans can also *act* on the basis of self-imposed maxims that "determine the human faculty of desire,"[138] provided that these maxims satisfy the criteria of rationality. Perhaps the most influential – and still dominant – theory on agency is the one that was formulated by Immanuel Kant. For him, agency and free will seem to be almost identical, the former being defined as

> a species of causality of living beings, insofar as they are rational, and freedom would be that quality of this causality by which it can be effective independently of alien causes determining it; just as natural necessity is the quality of the causality of all beings lacking reason, of being determined to activity through the influence of alien causes.[139]

The upshot is that only beings of rational nature, that is, humans, may act independently of natural necessity on their own free will and agency, the latter being understood by Kant as

> a special kind of causality, namely a causality that acts under normative principles, hence a capacity to choose between alternatives according to one's judgment about which alternative is permitted or required by a norm.[140]

---

[138] Valtteri Viljanen, "Kant on Moral Agency: Beyond the Incorporation Thesis," *Kant-Studien* 111, no. 3 (2020): 425.

[139] Immanuel Kant, *Groundwork for the Metaphysics of Morals*, ed. and trans. Allen W. Wood (New Haven, CT, and London: Yale University Press, 2002), 4:446.

[140] Allen W. Wood, "What is Kantian Ethics?" in Immanuel Kant, *Groundwork*

In view of the above, the faculty of rationality – which, as far as Kant is concerned, is unique to humans – may mediate our inclinations, and "although our faculty of desire can never remain untouched by ('impulsive') desires or inclinations, we are not at their mercy;"[141] on the contrary, "however they [our predispositions] may affect us, cannot determine our will unless they are incorporated into our maxims by our free power of choice."[142]

All the above may well explain why humans, now seen as rational moral agents who can act *for* or *towards* freely established ends, are different – and, maybe, in that sense unique – in comparison to every other species: Let us assume that indeed chipmunks do not seem capable of acting for or towards ends, although their actions sometimes look as if they were aimed either at some certain state of affairs, or at some other thing or individual. Even then, this can only tell us that humans are unique as a species, but in no case unique as particular individual beings: On the contrary, if all rational moral agents do act according to maxims that are imposed by reason, there is nothing irreplaceable or outstanding in each one of them, nothing to make each one of them unique. But this mostly concerns Kant's view on human dignity, which I intent to discuss later: What is it that makes individual moral agents irreplaceable, if to be a moral agent means to act on maxims that meet the criteria of reason, which in turn means that, since any maxim would either be accepted or rejected by reason, every rational moral agent would unavoidably act *on*

for the Metaphysics of Morals, ed. and trans. Allen W. Wood, 157-181 (New Haven, CT, and London: Yale University Press, 2002), 175.

[141] Viljanen, 424.

[142] John Rawls, *Lectures on the History of Moral Philosophy*, ed. Barbara Herman (Cambridge, MA: Harvard University Press, 2000), 295.

the same maxim? In any case, the creation of identical copies of rational moral agents doesn't seem to threaten the alleged uniqueness of the species *Homo sapiens* as standing out from all other species, nor would it seem capable of compromising the uniqueness of any individual human person, at least no more that the 'normal' birth of any newborn individual would.

iv. Incommunicability

It is true that each human being indeed does have certain qualities in common – as a matter of fact, *all* their qualities – with other individual beings, especially – but not only – with those who belong to the species *Homo sapiens*; nonetheless, there seems to be *something* that is incommunicably her own, that makes her "exist in some sense for [her] own sake, each existing as incommunicably her own,"[143] something that transcends her qualitatively or quantitatively explainable nature and cannot be accounted for:

> […] in a human being there is not only that human nature which he has in common with all other human beings, but also something that he has as his own – his own and not another's – incommunicably his own. Obviously, a human being would not amount to an individual being if he were not, over and above all that he has in common with others, also incommunicably his own.[144]

---

[143] John F. Crosby III, "The Incommunicability of Human Persons," *The Thomist: A Speculative Quarterly Review* 57, no. 3 (1993): 403.

[144] John F. Crosby III, "Why Persons Have Dignity," *Life and Learning IX: Proceedings of the Ninth University Faculty for Life Conference*, ed. Joseph W. Koterski, 79-92 (Washington DC: University Faculty for Life, 2000), 83.

Incommunicability, although reportedly[145] it is already mentioned as a concept in Roman law, where the person is defined as "sui juris et alteri incommunicabilis,"[146] i.e., as something that belongs to itself and does not share its being with another, denotes a concept that is very difficult to define, obscure in its vagueness: It is "the name of a way of being that is unique to a particular individual,"[147] and signifies "what is irreplaceable about a person,"[148] since it implies "that this person is not able to be repeated in some sense or other by the other persons."[149] As Crosby aptly points out, what is incommunicable in each of us justifies lamenting the deceased,[150] for when a person pass-

---

[145] Despite the unanimity of scholars on this, the phrase is not actually present in the Roman Law as such. It seems possible that it was coined by the early medieval scholastics to crystallize concepts that are indeed present in the roman though. In his *Instutiones* Gaius draws the line between persons that are *sui iuris*, and those who are in *alienam potestatem* (Gaii Instituones, liber I, 78); see *Institutes of Roman Law by Gaius*, trans. Edward Poste, rev. E.A. Whittuck (Oxford: Clarendon Press, 1904), book I, art. 78ff.

[146] As cited by Crosby, "The Uniqueness of Persons," 408. To Aquinas, "Hoc nomen persona significat substantiam particularem, prout subjicitur proprietati quae sonat Dignitatem," Aquinas, *Commentary on the Sentences of Peter Lombard*, book 1, distinction 23, article 1, as cited in Marek Piechowiak, "Thomas Aquinas – Human Dignity and Conscience as a Basis for Restricting Legal Obligations," *Diametros* 47 (2016): 71. As to the incommunicability of persons, Aquinas postulates that: "the very meaning of person is that it is incommunicable" (licet persona sit incommunicabilis, tamen ipse modus existendi incommunicabiliter, potest esse pluribus communis), Aquinas, *Summa Theologica*, book I, question 30, article 4, objection 2. See also Karol Wojtyla, "The Personal Structure of Self-Determination," in Karol Wojtyla, *Person and Act and Related Essays*, trans. Grzegorz Ignatik (Washington DC: Catholic University of America Press, 2021), 192-193.

[147] Zagzebski, "The Uniqueness of Persons," 414.

[148] Ibid., 415.

[149] Crosby, "The Incommunicability of Human Persons," 405.

[150] Ibid., 404.

es away, something unrepeatable in her is lost forever, something that cannot be compensated for by the characteristics and qualities of other people that continue to live around us.

The concept of incommunicability puts the emphasis on what distinguishes individual beings from each other. But it is also a fact that there is no quality or characteristic that any individual being does not share with other beings, and this inevitably blurs the distinction: The *humanity* of each individual human being, for example, in light of the above is incommunicably her own, and that makes one absolutely distinguishable as standing out against all others of one's kind, but at the same time unites all in a way that makes it sensible to refer to each distinct individual as a 'human being.' I tend to think of *my* humanity as incommunicably *my own*, but that humanity of mine is also a quality I share with all other human beings, *even in the sense that it is incommunicably my own*: What makes us all humans is the property of humanity, but this humanity of ours is incommunicably one's own for each one of us. Could there be a way out of the conundrum? Crosby suggests that we should distinguish between the *thick* and the *thin* sense of properties such as humanity, that seem to distinguish and unite individual beings as communicable and incommunicable at the same time, or, as he puts it, between the *concrete* and the *general idea* of properties as such. In that sense,

> The communicability of humanity […] would lie primarily in the general idea; humanity does not coincide with anyone's concrete humanity but in some sense transcends all human beings so as to be able to be common to them all […]. In other words, that which results in a being through its participating in some universal or some commu-

> nicable idea, that limiting of and reducing of its
> incommunicable selfhood, can be called a kind
> of concrete communicability. In fact, we will usu-
> ally be speaking of communicable being in this
> more concrete sense. It follows that the humanity
> of Socrates is communicable in one respect, and
> incommunicable in another. It is communica-
> ble in the secondary sense just explained, but it
> is incommunicable insofar as it is Socrates' own
> and is therefore to be distinguished from Plato's
> humanity.[151]

This opens a new perspective on why persons and only persons are incommunicable to others: Persons exist as *real* individual beings, and all real beings, as such, can only be the beings they are, and not any other of their kind, otherwise they
would dissolve into the general idea in which they participate.
Persons, in particular, unlike mere 'natures,' do have a self, and
their incommunicability lies precisely in their selfhood, since
this "incommunicable selfhood which is proper to every being
is raised, in personal being, to a higher power."[152] So, while
non-persons are also incommunicable, there is something in
the incommunicability of persons that elevates them above
any other being: We are justified in being more interested in
the incommunicability of a particular human person, for example, than in the incommunicability of a particular rock; the
combined fact of life and consciousness is, according to Crosby, what justifies regarding the general incommunicability of
persons as stronger than that of other, non-personal instances
of nature:

---

[151] Ibid., 408.

[152] Ibid., 409.

> Consider a copy of today's newspaper, of which, we will assume, millions of copies have been printed. Any copy is of course incommunicably itself and is not any other. But notice that it is unreasonable to take any interest in the incommunicable being of the one copy; whatever interests me in the one copy would interest me equally in any other copy; no one copy has anything which I could not as well find in any other copy. The incommunicable being of each copy exists entirely for the sake of that which is common to them ; it is there only for the sake of instantiating and multiplying the communicable […]. The incommunicability which we find in human persons, however, is incomparable with any order of being below the person. In the realm of our direct experience it is the human person which forms the most extreme antithesis to the specimen-being of each copy of the newspaper […].[153]

In the personalist view, human persons – unlike rocks and newspaper copies – are not subject to the laws of numerical quantity, and this is why the *sorites paradox* is not applicable to persons: A person is not simply *less* than two – or two million – persons, just as it is not simply *more* than none; this explains the intuitive thought that a person cannot simply be replaced by another, as grains of wheat, or rocks, or newspaper copies can: If someone, in my absence, replaced a grain or all the grains in the heap with exactly the same number of grains and arranged them in exactly the same shape, I wouldn't be able to determine that *this* heap is not the heap

---

[153] Ibid., 410-412.

I first saw. Replacing grains with others would simply make no difference. With persons, on the other hand, it does make a difference, and that is why we love certain persons and mourn them when they pass away, even though their qualities are also common to other persons. Strictly speaking, each individual person is irreplaceable, since "he has personhood as so incommunicably his own that, though he is not the only person, he nevertheless 'appears in being' as if he were the only one."[154] To appear *as if being the only one* means that, whereas in the case of the grains of wheat one might rightly assume that adding or removing them would lead only to quantitative differentiations in the heap, the existence of each person *qua person* does not simply add to the number of existing persons; rather, each person seems to constitute *its own numerical infinity*, which adds itself infinitely to every other person, and at the same time paradoxically adds nothing, because each person is a numerical infinity in itself, and to that which is infinite nothing can be added; in Guardini's words, the person "is the fact that it exists in the form of belonging to oneself."[155]

The fact that human persons do not exist as mere specimens of humanity suffices to elevate them above the qualitative and quantitative manifestations of value; rather, it is this incommunicable selfhood of human persons that justifies regarding each of them as infinitely valuable: "Now for the first time the value datum which we call the dignity of the human person would appear, and it would appear as rooted in incommunicable selfhood."[156] In Crosby's personalist view the concept of incommunicability is interwoven with that of dignity, i.e., the fact that "persons already have a certain infinite worth in virtue of simply being persons."[157] This

---

[154] Ibid., 414.

[155] Roman Guardini, *The World and the Person*, trans. Stella Lange (Chicago: Henry Regnery, 1965), 118.

[156] Crosby, "The Incommunicability of Human Persons," 429.

[157] Ibid., 431.

incommunicable personhood of the human being is the primary ground for human dignity.[158]

The view that only humans exist as something more than mere specimens of their species sounds convincing enough when humans are weighed against, say, goldfish: Goldfish seem to be interchangeable specimens, and indeed it makes no sense to mourn the loss of the *one* goldfish that has just died in its bowl. But once we move from goldfish to dogs, Crosby's view is on shaky ground: Odysseus, we believe, had perfectly good reasons to mourn the loss of his dog, Argos, who was by no means replaceable for him as a mere specimen of a dog. Had *you* not mourned the loss of the dog you lived with, your friends would at best consider you an uncaring, insensitive person – and nobody would blame them for this. I remain unconvinced that dignity, if it 'is rooted in incommunicable selfhood,' should be reserved only for humans – but that is the subject of another book. To return to the subject of this book: So far, at any rate, we have not found a conclusive argument against human cloning on the basis that it challenges the assumed uniqueness of human beings; indeed, we have not even succeeded in establishing the concept of uniqueness as a special property of human beings. The only clue we seem to be left with is the assumed link between human uniqueness and human dignity.

c. From incommunicability to dignity

The concept of dignity is "notoriously vague"[159] and overwhelmingly elusive; it also stubbornly resists any attempt at philosophical definition. But there is at least a trail we can follow if we pick

---

[158] Crosby, "Why Persons Have Dignity," 10. See also, Stephen L. Brock, "Is Uniqueness at the Root of Personal Dignity? John Crosby and Thomas Aquinas," *The Thomist* 69 (2005): 174.

[159] David Gurnham, "The Mysteries of Human Dignity and the Brave New World of Human Cloning," *Social and Legal Studies* 14, no. 2 (2005): 199.

up where we left off in the previous chapter: It is almost a com-monplace that dignity is closely associated with uniqueness. We are inclined to think that anything that has dignity must necessarily be unique for that reason, and that anything that is not unique cannot have dignity. But this is not always true in re-verse: Anything that is unique does not necessarily have dignity for that reason – while dignity necessarily implies uniqueness, uniqueness does not necessarily imply dignity. If it is true that uniqueness is at the root of dignity, then surely a certain kind of uniqueness is needed to serve as the basis for dignity. On the question of what that kind of uniqueness is, Crosby's account is in my view the most inclusive, and for that reason probably one with the strongest initial appeal: For him the ground of dignity is his version of uniqueness, which he calls *incommunicability*, and which applies only to persons.

To reach this conclusion Crosby first distinguishes be-tween four types of incommunicability. The first one is [a] "not being predicable of many,"[160] but this kind of incommunicabili-ty does not confer any particular value – not to speak of dignity, since it indicates a kind of uniqueness that is "merely numer-ical, […] not formal, 'being one of a kind'"[161]: The individual human being does not differ from other individual creatures in 'not being predicable of many.' But even this [b] 'being one of a kind' type of incommunicability would not be sufficient to es-tablish dignity: As Crosby aptly notes, being the last dinosaur or the only daughter of the Smiths is no indication of any special worth or value, all the more so because uniqueness – or, incom-municability – in this respect can only be absolutely *incidental*, and says nothing about a creature's intrinsic worth or inherent

---

[160] John F. Crosby, *The Selfhood of the Human Person* (Washington DC: The Catholic University of America Press, 1996), 46.

[161] Stephen Brock, 175.

value. Incommunicability is also not [c] about "some intrinsic value, that would be at least practically impossible to repeat, but that pertain only to the realm of abilities, achievements, and so forth."[162] The marvelous achievements of Alexander the Great during his lifetime, say, are not sufficient to establish his value as existing for his own sake – they can only prove the value of his qualities or deeds. What is needed here is something else: "the value pertaining to the very subject, the person herself, in her sheer 'selfhood.'"[163] So Crosby says:

> In our new personalist perspective, it would not only be qualities and excellences but rather also the subject of them, the one who has them, this or that particular human being, which would stand before us as worthy, good. Now for the first time the value datum called the dignity of the human person would appear, and it would appear as rooted in incommunicable selfhood.[164]

For Crosby, unlike other living things, plants, or animals, human persons have an *inner center* that is "immeasurably richer and deeper,"[165] what Newman calls the "unfathomable depth," or the "infinite abyss of existence,"[166] and this infinity "seems almost to coincide with personal incommunicability [since each person is] so strong a being of his own that he exists as if in a sense the others did not exist."[167]

---

[162] Ibid., 176.

[163] Ibid.

[164] Crosby, *The Selfhood of the Human Person*, 66.

[165] Stephen Brock, 177.

[166] See John Henry Newman, "The Individuality of the Soul," *Parochial and Plain Sermons* (San Francisco: Ignatius Press, 1997), 784-792.

[167] Stephen Brock, 178.

> Each person exists 'as if there were no other,' 'as if he or she were the only one,' etc. This would be the special incommunicability or uniqueness that is proper to persons, and which, unlike the other types of uniqueness, would match with their personal dignity: to exist as if there were no other.[168]

It is this unrepeatable and incommunicable *selfhood* of persons, the fact that each person exists *as if he or she were the only one* and all else "live in his light" in the expression of Martin Buber,[169] that constitutes human dignity. In my view Crosby's account permeates – and is consonant with – all theories of human dignity as their backbone from Boethius to Immanuel Kant, regardless of any differences in their approach, views, or focus.

d. Distinctiveness "by reason of dignity"

Our contemporary notion of dignity is that of an "unearned, distinctive, inalienable human value, […] a universal and inalienable property of human beings, which can serve as the foundation of basic human rights."[170] What makes each human being distinctive to any other member of her species and all other creatures is that, since she exists as if she were the only one, that is, an unrepeatable, incommunicable person, it may only be immensely infinite as the person she is, in such

---

[168] Ibid.

[169] Martin Buber, *I and Thou* (New York: Charles Scribner's Sons, 1958), 100, as quoted in Stephen Brock, 178.

[170] Miriam Griffin, "Dignity in Roman and Stoic Thought," in *Dignity: A History*, ed. Remy Debes, 47-65 (New York: Oxford University Press, 2017), 47-48.

a way as adding to it would add nothing to the whole, and removing it would remove everything. In the words of Seneca persons have *genuine merit*, i.e., dignity, while everything else may have some value: Unlike persons, they exist for the sake of another, and they are subject to numerical, that is, qualitative or quantitative, differentiation:

> Bodily goods are, to be sure, good for the body; but they are not absolutely good. There will indeed be some value [*pretium*] in them; but they will possess no genuine merit [*dignitas*], for they will differ greatly; some will be less, others greater.[171]

Human persons, on the other hand, are exalted above all price, according to the famous phrase of Immanuel Kant, because they possess dignity:

> In the realm of ends everything has either a price or a dignity. What has a price is such that something else can also be put in its place as its equivalent; by contrast, that which is elevated above all price, and admits of no equivalent, has a dignity.[172]

Kant does nothing here but follow the same strand with Thomas Aquinas; Aquinas quotes and favors Alan of Lille's definition of a

---

[171] "Corporum autem bona corporibus quidem bona sunt, sed in totum non sunt bona. His pretium quidem erit aliquod, ceterum dignitas non erit; magnis inter se intervallis distabunt; alia minora, alia maiora erunt." Seneca, "Epistle LXXI.," 33-34, in *Ad Lucilum epistulae morales*, ed. and trans. Richard Gummere (Cambridge, MA: Harvard University Press).

[172] Kant, *Groundwork for the Metaphysics of Morals*, 4:443.

person: "A person is a substance distinct by reason of dignity."[173] Again, the idea of human uniqueness – in terms of Crosby's incommunicability – can be seen as reinforcing and strengthening the notion of human dignity by emphasizing the special qualities that make human beings so special and valuable that they 'admit of no equivalent.' Kant further elucidates his view by always following the path paved by Seneca and distinguishing between market price, affective price, and dignity:

> That which refers to universal human inclinations and needs has a market price; that which, even without presupposing any need, is in accord with a certain taste, i.e., a satisfaction in the mere purposeless play of the powers of our mind, an affective price; but that which constitutes the condition under which alone something can be an end in itself does not have merely a relative worth, i.e., a price, but rather an inner worth, i.e., dignity.[174]

It is clear that the way Kant conceives of dignity – nothing 'can also be put in its place as its equivalent,' while it 'does not have merely a relative worth' – implies that to have dignity is to be *irreplaceable* on the one hand and *infinitely valuable* on the other, and that both are true at the same time. The result is that dignity makes one incomparably valuable, even in relation to other beings who are also accorded dignity. In Zagzebski's words:

> Kant's discussion of a dignity implies two different things. One is that anything that has dignity

---

[173] Aquinas, *Summa Theologica*, book I, question 29, article 3, reply to objection 2: "Persona est hypostasis proprietate distincta ad dignitatem pertinente."

[174] Kant, *Groundwork for the Metaphysics of Morals*, 4:434-435.

is more valuable than any number of things that have a price, no matter how high the price. The other is that things with dignity cannot be compared in value to anything else, not even to other things with dignity. That means we can never make up for the loss of a thing with dignity by replacing it with another or even many others. Kant apparent1y thought that the two aspects of dignity – infinite value and irreplaceable value – must go together.[175]

For Kant it is true that dignity, i.e. being irreplaceable and infinitely valuable –Zagzebski believes that these two concepts, although not identical, for Kant they are logically connected – is reserved only for 'humanity and every rational nature,'[176] which for Kant is practically the same thing.[177] This is because, for Kant, dignity cannot be thought of in any other way but as dependent on – and presupposing – rationality, that allows human beings, i.e., rational moral agents, to break free from the laws of natural heteronomy (when the imperative is conditioned by "an object of the will [that] must be taken as the ground in order to describe the rule determining that will")[178] and to enjoy what he calls 'freedom of the will,' which for him is "autonomy, i.e., the quality of the will of being a law to itself."[179] In a word, according to Kant, dignity, that is, "unconditioned, incomparable worth," is intrinsically – better, *causally* – related to rationality and autonomy:

---

[175] Zagzebski, "The Uniqueness of Persons," 402.

[176] See, for example, Kant, *Groundwork for the Metaphysics of Morals*, 4:430, and 4:436, where Kant discusses autonomy.

[177] Here I fully endorse Allen Wood's view; see Kant, *Groundwork for the Metaphysics of Morals*, note 63 on page 47.

[178] Kant, *Groundwork for the Metaphysics of Morals*, 4:444.

[179] Ibid., 4:447.

> The legislation itself, however, which determines all
> worth, must precisely for this reason have a digni-
> ty, i.e., an unconditioned, incomparable worth; the
> word respect alone yields a becoming expression
> for the estimation that a rational being must assign
> to it. Autonomy is thus the ground of the dignity of
> the human and of every rational nature.[180]

Kant's view is consistent with Boethius' previously discussed
definition of personhood, as well as Aquinas' aphorism that
"person signifies what is most perfect in all of nature, that is, a
subsistent individual of a rational nature."[181] In summary, according to this line of thought, which begins with Boethius,
culminates with Kant, and crystallizes in Crosby, because only
persons are of a rational nature, only persons can be incommunicable, and this is what gives them their dignity – this boils
down to that what can have dignity is a being with a rational
nature. It is in this respect that persons are distinguished from
every other being in creation – as infinitely and incomparably
valuable – 'by reason of their dignity.'

e. Personal and impersonal dignity

The concept of dignity is a slippery one, and this is evident from
the fact that it can apply equally to persons who presently exist,

---

[180] Ibid., 4:436.

[181] Aquinas, *Summa Theologica*, Part I, Question 29, Article 3: "Respondeo
dicendum quod persona significat id quod est perfectissimum in tota
natura, scilicet subsistens in rationali natura." For an excellent discussion
on personhood and dignity see Gilles Emery, "The Dignity of Being a
Substance: Person, Subsistence, and Nature," *Nova et Vetera* 9, no. 4 (2011):
991-1001.

but also to those who have died or do not yet exist: We can comfortably talk about *my* dignity or *your* dignity, but we can also talk about the dignity of the dead and of future generations, or – within the context of certain worldviews – about the dignity of the fertilized egg and the embryo. You and I are, of course, persons, insofar as we are – at least in the light of the Kantian tradition – rational beings; future generations, the dead, and embryos, on the other hand, are not. This implies, according to Dieter Birnbacher, that there is "no unitary and homogeneous concept of human dignity, but rather a family of meanings in the Wittgensteinian sense, the members of which behave differently not only semantically but also syntactically."[182] Birnbacher distinguishes between two types of dignity, *personal* and *impersonal*: While the concept of personal dignity is applicable to individual persons – because it necessarily "presupposes an individual bearer,"[183] impersonal dignity refers to the species *Homo sapiens* as a whole, and in this sense dignity can also refer to future generations as well as to non-persons such as human corpses or embryos. Birnbacher believes that dignity can only be explained in a personal sense as a kind of moral right. I assume that he does not mean that the concept of dignity *itself* can be regarded as a moral right, but that various rights can be regarded as connected to or based on dignity, in the sense that the dignity of the moral person is affected when these rights are violated.

Birnbacher further distinguishes between two meanings attributed to human dignity in the personal sense, a *central* one, in which dignity can be conceived as a constellation of moral rights that impose negative and positive duties on others, and

---

[182] Dieter Birnbacher, "Human Cloning and Human Dignity," *Reproductive BioMedicine Online* 10, Supplement 1 (2005): 51.
[183] Ibid.

in this sense respecting a person's dignity primarily means not treating her merely as a means to an end, and another, a *marginal* one, in which the concept of dignity implies a certain moral status.[184] In its central meaning dignity,

> is typically the dignity of the victim, [while] individual human dignity in its marginal use is typically the dignity of the trespasser. In violations of human dignity, both, as it were, have their dignity compromised, the victim by being treated in a way a human being should not be treated by virtue of his humanity, the trespasser by treating others (or himself) in a way a human being should not do in virtue of his humanity.[185]

With impersonal, *generic* dignity, on the other hand, there can be perpetrators, but no victims: A corpse, as an impersonal form of human existence, cannot become a victim, but the dignity of humanity can be violated through it if the corpse is treated merely as a means to an end: Destroying a corpse for experimental purposes or 'degrading' it in some way may do nothing to the corpse itself, but it would constitute a violation of human dignity in the person of the perpetrator in an impersonal sense – if this seems very Kantian to you, you are probably right. "The harm which is done in these cases," Birnbacher aptly notes, "is largely or exclusively symbolic harm, like the harm done by blasphemy."[186] There always seems, of course, to be some connection between the disregard of non-personal

---

[184] On this, see also Peonidis' "deflationary account" of human dignity; Filimon Peonidis, "Making Sense of Dignity: A Starting Point," *Conatus – Journal of Philosophy* 5, no. 1 (2020): 85-100.

[185] Birnbacher, 51.

[186] Ibid., 53.

and personal dignity, so that one can rightly assume that the disregard of the former prepares the ground for the disregard of the latter, or, as Kant would put it, disrespecting human dignity in a corpse

> is far more intimately opposed to man's duty to himself, and he has a duty to refrain from this; for it dulls his shared feeling [...] and so weakens and gradually uproots a natural predisposition that is very serviceable to morality in one's relations with other men.[187]

The fact remains, however, that dignity in its generic sense entails a very different set of obligations than dignity in its personal sense. There also remains the question of the extent to which human reproductive cloning would affect human dignity in either sense. Birnbacher argues that cloning does not pose a threat to either, at least not a significant one or one that does not also emanate from natural reproduction, and I am inclined to agree wholeheartedly with his view: Instrumentalization, reification, paternalism, and other threats as such to human dignity in its personal form, "are only contingently related to cloning, they are not inherent to it,"[188] whereas I really cannot see how the idea or the process of human cloning itself could be considered a violation of human dignity in its generic, impersonal form, unless there were some truly bizarre genetic engineering at play, aimed at creating chimeras whose existence would threaten the dignity we so readily ascribe to our species; but again, this would be a legitimate concern against this bizarre

---

[187] Immanuel Kant, *Metaphysics of Morals*, trans. Mary Gregor (Cambridge: Cambridge University Press, 1991), 6:443.

[188] Birnbacher, 51.

application of genetic engineering, but in no sense a legitimate concern against human cloning.

But again, if human dignity is understood as a 'constellation of moral rights' or, better, as the basis of a set of rights, human reproductive cloning could violate not the concept of dignity itself in its personal or impersonal sense, but instead certain rights that are based on dignity; in other words, human dignity could also be violated in an indirect way by disregarding what it produces or generates.

f. Human dignity as the ground of rights

What we generally call *moral rights* correspond more or less to *moral freedoms*, that is, *permissions* for the moral agent to act or not to act in a certain way. A woman's moral right to abortion, for example, gives her the freedom to choose whether to maintain or terminate her pregnancy. Duties, on the other hand, represent a *voluntary restriction* on our moral freedom: If I believe that I have a moral duty to tell the truth to someone who asks me for information, then I do not have the moral freedom to lie – *I ought to tell the truth.* Of course, I always have the discretion not to fulfill that duty and lie. But then I would be violating the right of my fellow human beings to the truth, and influential moral philosophers at various times have given a variety of reasons why I should not do so.

In any case, a connection between the concept of a right and that of a duty is evident in such a way that either the recognition of a right entails corresponding duties of other moral persons towards the holder of that right, or, conversely, the recognition of a duty for the moral person gives rise to corresponding rights for other moral persons.

> To say that A has a "right" that B not do X to A is
> to say that B has a "duty" not to do X to A; to say

that A has a "right" that B do Y for A is to say that
B has a "duty" to do Y for A.[189]

In its first version, this two-way relationship seems to impose
negative duties on the environment of the moral agent who
is the bearer of a particular right. In other words, if a person
possesses the right to the free expression of her opinion, her
environment has a corresponding duty *not to* impose restrictions on that person's ability to express herself freely. To the
extent that a right is expected to give rise to a corresponding
negative duty, i.e., to create a *prohibition*, the recognition of
rights for moral persons seems to constitute an effective way
of protecting them against undesirable and potentially negative situations.

Given that the debate over human reproductive cloning
is currently framed in terms of securing certain minimum
guarantees – as is the case with any scientific innovation that
significantly changes our lives and perceptions – it is not surprising that much of the ethical debate over cloning revolves
around the notion of human rights and moral personhood.
Some argue that cloning is a way to secure or promote certain
moral rights, or that stopping its development and not legalizing its use would be a violation of some of those rights. Others
argue that morally legitimizing human reproductive cloning
and then legalizing it would inevitably lead to the violation of
some of those rights.

To start from this last point: If there is a right to freedom
of scientific research, then any interference aimed at stopping
scientific progress in human reproductive cloning would seem
to violate that right. Conversely, if every human being has the

[189] Michael J. Perry, "The Morality of Human Rights," *San Diego Law Review*
50, no. 4 (2013): 777.

right to reproduce herself and to choose freely the manner of her reproduction, then cloning seems to protect this right. On the contrary, human reproductive cloning seems to violate the human right to uniqueness – whether genotypic, phenotypic, or any other form – to the extent that cloning is a method of creating genetic copies. Similarly, human cloning appears to violate the right of the resulting clone to be unaware of her genetic nature and future, and the corresponding right to potentially infinite realization in her life, usually referred to as the right to an open future. Of the above rights that are either promoted or impaired by cloning, the first two, freedom of scientific research and procreation, are traditional rights – in the sense that they are not being introduced for the first time in the context of the cloning debate. The right to an open future was first introduced by Joel Feinberg in relation to minors whose future options are deliberately limited by their environment, but the cloning debate seems to serve as the right environment for this right to develop to its full potential. The right to uniqueness and the corresponding right to genetic ignorance constitute new arguments that their proponents propose as necessary determinants for the ethical debate on cloning. In what follows, I will discuss these concerns in terms of their relevance to the concept of dignity, either as a means of enhancing or eliminating it.

2. Human Dignity and Human Reproductive Cloning

A brief look at statements and opinions of all kinds from international and professional bodies is sufficient to show that the almost unanimous skepticism – if not outright rejection – of human reproductive cloning is based in large part on concerns about the threat to human dignity that it might pose. These concerns are primarily based on the alleged dependence of human dignity on a trait that can only be demonstrated in humans, namely their uniqueness, which reproductive cloning is supposed to call into question. Both, however, need to be thoroughly debated: Are there good reasons to believe that human dignity does indeed depend on uniqueness, and if so, does cloning actually pose a threat to this precious uniqueness of the human being?

The first resolution by an international body on human reproductive cloning was that of the World Health Organization on May 14, 1997, and it appears to affirm these two questions:

> Recognizing that developments in cloning and other genetic procedures have unprecedented ethical implications and considering that related research and development should therefore be carefully monitored and assessed, and the rights and dignity of patients respected, 1. Affirms that the use of cloning for the replication of human individuals is ethically unacceptable and contrary to human integrity and morality.[190]

[190] World Health Organization, "Cloning in Human Reproduction," World Health Assembly, 50.37, 1997, https://apps.who.int/iris/

A few months later, on November 11, 1997, the WHO resolution was reaffirmed by a Universal Declaration adopted by
UNESCO:

> Practices which are contrary to human dignity,
> such as reproductive cloning of human beings,
> shall not be permitted. States and competent in-
> ternational organizations are invited to cooper-
> ate in identifying such practices and in taking,
> at national or international level, the measures
> necessary to ensure that the principles set out in
> this Declaration are respected.[191]

On May 16, 1998, the World Health Organization came back
with a more detailed statement, calling for a worldwide ban on
human reproductive cloning on grounds of protecting human
dignity:

> 1. Reaffirms that cloning for the replication of
> human individuals is ethically unacceptable and
> contrary to human dignity and integrity.
> 2. Urges Member States to foster continued and
> informed debate on these issues and to take ap-
> propriate steps, including legal and juridical
> measures, to prohibit cloning for the purpose of
> replicating human individuals.[192]

---

handle/10665/179791.

[191] UNESCO, "Universal Declaration on the Human Genome and Human
Rights," in *Records of the General Conference. Volume 1: Resolutions*, 41-46
(Paris: UNESCO, 1998), Article 11.

[192] World Health Organization, "Ethical, scientific and social implications
of cloning in human health," World Health Assembly, 51.10, 1998, https://

In 1998, the Council of Europe issued an Additional Protocol. What is new about this protocol, is that it associates human replication with the risk of instrumentalization:

> The instrumentalization of human beings through the deliberate creation of genetically identical human beings is contrary to human dignity and thus constitutes a misuse of biology and medicine. 1. Any intervention seeking to create a human being genetically identical to another human being, whether living or dead, is prohibited. 2. For the purpose of this article, the term human being "genetically identical" to another human being means a human being sharing with another the same nuclear gene set.[193]

It is clear in all these statements that they deal with human reproductive cloning on the basis of *principles*, not on the basis of *risks and benefits*; cloning is discussed as *prima facie* evil, a *malum ad se*, rather than as a *malum prohibitum*. Thus, from the outset, concerns about the actual consequences of cloning for the prototype and the clone are left out of the debate: What should be addressed first is whether cloning might be compatible with 'human morality,' as the WHO's resolution puts it. According to Dieter Birnbacher,

> As a rule, this judgement is taken to imply a particularly strong moral condemnation, and, fur-

---

apps.who.int/iris/handle/10665/79804.

[193] Council of Europe, *Additional Protocol to the Convention for the Protection of Human Rights and Dignity of the Human Being with regard to the Application of Biology and Medicine, on the Prohibition of Cloning Human Beings* (Paris: Council of Europe, 1998).

thermore, one that is categorical and independent of consequences. The intuition underlying
the judgement seems to be that reproductive
cloning is in itself a violation of human dignity,
and that it should not be attempted even if we
were certain that it could be done without serious risks to the potential clone, its environment
and society at large.[194]

As I indicated in the chapter entitled 'Norms and Principles,'
invoking principles is the first line of defense for bioethics
against potentially dangerous innovations, such as human reproductive cloning; we might also think of principles as the
first of two necessary filters that something must pass through
before it is accepted, the second being the actual consequences for those affected. This second filter, however, may only be
reached if the innovation under discussion has successfully
passed the first filter, i.e., its compatibility with moral principles. The moral argument that the statements and resolutions
I have cited above boil down to, is the following:

> A. Any artificial intervention aimed at creating two or
> more human beings with the same nuclear gene set vio-
> lates human dignity, integrity, and morality.
> B. Anything that violates human dignity results in the
> instrumentalization of human beings.
> C. Human reproductive cloning aims to produce two
> or more human beings with the same nuclear gene set.
> D. Therefore, human reproductive cloning violates hu-
> man dignity, integrity and morality, resulting thus in
> the instrumentalization of human beings.

---

[194] Birnbacher, 50. See also Malby, 103.

Here I will only attempt to discuss and clarify the key concepts on which the argument is based; in subsequent chapters I will discuss all its implications in detail. I must say at the outset, however, that of the premises only the second seems to me to be prima facie true, but in that case, it may just be the Kantian in me talking. I realize that not everyone agrees with the view that there is a necessary connection between human dignity and instrumentalization, such that anyone who is instrumentalized necessarily gives up their own dignity; moreover, I am also aware of the fact that many are skeptical of the concept of human dignity itself,[195] or of limiting dignity only to human beings.[196] Nevertheless, I will assume for the purposes of this discussion that there is indeed such a quality in human beings as dignity, and that this quality is of as much importance as it is commonly accorded. For the purposes of this discussion,

---

[195] For Schopenhauer, dignity is "nothing but a hollow hyperbole, within which there lurks like a gnawing worm, *contradictio in adjecto*." Arthur Schopenhauer, *The Basis of Morality* (London, and Aylesbury: Hazell, Wattson and Viney, 1903), 101. For an excellent discussion see Marián Palenčár, "Some Remarks on the Concept and Intellectual History of Human Dignity," *Human Affairs* 26 (2016): 462-477; also Marcus Düwell, "Human Dignity: Concepts, Discussions, Philosophical Perspectives," in *The Cambridge Handbook of Human Dignity*, eds. M. Düwell, J. Braarvig, R. Brownsword, and D. Mieth, 23-49 (Cambridge: Cambridge University Press, 2014).

[196] Nussbaum, among others, has called for the concept of dignity to be expanded to include non-human animals. In her view dignity is an "animal sort of dignity, and that very sort of dignity could not be possessed by a being who was not mortal and vulnerable, just as the beauty of a cherry tree in bloom could not be possessed by a diamond." See Martha Nussbaum, *Frontiers of Justice: Disability, Nationality, Species Membership* (Cambridge, MA: Harvard University Press, 2006), 132. See, also, Federico Zuolo, "Dignity and Animals. Does it Make Sense to Apply the Concept of Dignity to all Sentient Beings?" *Ethical Theory and Moral Practice* 19 (2016): 1-13.

it seems unnecessary to me to explore whether beings other than humans could share in this property. I will also assume that the concepts of instrumentalization and dignity are indeed incompatible, so that any violation of dignity necessarily leads to the instrumentalization of the being whose dignity is being disregarded, and conversely, any being that is considered merely as a means to an end necessarily lacks the property of dignity. Having commented on these points, I may now proceed to some necessary clarifications on the key concept of the argument against human reproductive cloning.

What the argument implies is that human dignity is somehow linked to uniqueness, and that 'being unique' should in turn be understood as 'having a unique nuclear gene set': As the Council of Europe puts it in the Additional Protocol quoted above, "the term […] 'genetically identical' […] means a human being sharing with another the same nuclear gene set."[197] Indeed, from the wording of the statements I have quoted it appears that what violates human dignity is "the replication of human individuals," or the "deliberate creation of genetically identical human beings." Here, then, one might think that if the only condition for possessing dignity were simply to be a human being, clones – since they would be identical copies of human beings, and thus human beings themselves – should be accorded that property as well; unless the property of dignity is reserved for 'human beings with a unique nuclear gene set,' and not merely for 'human beings.'

Such a view, though, could also exclude identical twins from the realm of dignity. Probably this is why all the above statements emphasize the *artificial* character of cloning – in contrast to the spontaneous, natural splitting of a zygote, which also produces two distinct human beings, who share

---

[197] Council of Europe.

the same nuclear gene set.[198] However, introducing such a pre-condition into the debate does not make the moral rejection of human reproductive cloning any more meaningful: Are there good reasons to believe that there are two distinct categories of 'clones' that differ in dignity only because of the way they were created – artificially or naturally? Is there something special about deliberate artificial interventions in general, that makes them incompatible with dignity? After all, artificial insemination is also a 'deliberate, artificial intervention' that results in a new human being that could not have existed without it, but no one today claims that in vitro fertilized zygotes result in human beings deprived of their dignity.[199] Thus, it should be neither the deliberate and artificial nature of the intervention, nor the fact that it will result in two human beings who share the same nucleus, but the combination of these two factors that can lead to the violation of human dignity. Still, the argument appears intuitively vague, and in need of good reasons.

There is also some ambiguity about what it is meant by the term 'creation of a human being.' At first glance,

> This is taken to mean a born human being, which excludes discussion on the ethics and human rights of technologies such as therapeutic cloning. The primary aim and result of HRC is procreation. Hence, this article artificially assumes that, after the intervention, the resulting human embryo is implanted and develops to full term without encountering any problems.[200]

---

[198] Malby, 104.

[199] Birmbacher, 53.

[200] Malby, 105.

Indeed, the cloning of individual human cells, tissues, and embryos for purposes other than implantation in a uterus and gestation seems irrelevant here. However, this means that the dignity that is violated in the case of human reproductive cloning is not the dignity of the donor of the genetic material, but the dignity of the human being created by this process. So, the question should be: Why should this 'intentional artificial intervention' aimed at creating a new living human being who shares 'the same core gene set' with an already existing person constitute a violation of that person's dignity? Again, we are in need of good reasons. There are, in fact, only two serious alternatives to be considered, to establish the conclusion that human reproductive cloning violates human dignity: Either the clone's dignity is violated by her being born as a clone, or the dignity of the human species as a whole is compromised in the face of the clone, due to the fact that she was born a clone. Neither of these possibilities, however, can be clearly conceived and maintained by those who oppose human reproductive cloning because, in their view, it violates human dignity: Once again in this case, those who endorse either one of these views, or both, would have to provide good reasons why we should not equally assume that the dignity of the individual, or that of the human species as a whole, or both, is not affected at all by the spontaneous, natural creation of homozygous twins.

A final point to discuss is the explicit reference to 'the same nuclear gene set' that is present in the resolutions I have quoted. The reason why nuclear genetic material deserves this special mention is probably because what human reproductive cloning is capable of producing is two *identical nuclei*, but by no means two *completely identical* genomes, for reasons I have already explained: The mitochondrial DNA can only be different, and however small this difference may be, it is still a reason to speak of merely *very similar* or *nearly identical* individuals. However, the fact remains that in the case of the clone and her prototype there is only nuclear identification, while in the case of homozygous twins – the closest case to that of clones – the mitochondrial DNA is also the same; yet, the dignity of identical twins is by no means debated, while that of clones is. The way I see it, the only way to make this distinction meaningful is to base it again on the fact that, in the case of cloning, the creation of new human beings, the clones, is due to this 'artificial intervention' that I mentioned earlier. But then, the question of in vitro fertilization and pre-implantation genetic engineering comes back on stage.

Up to this point, I have attempted to present the argument against human reproductive cloning in some detail, highlighting some of the concepts on which it is based and which I believe need clarification, and setting out only in outline some plausible objections that arise from it. In the following chapters of this book, I will discuss its implications in detail, and challenge it from various points of view, focusing on certain rights that seem to be sensitive either in the case of acceptance of human reproductive cloning or in the case of its rejection.

I. Advancing scientific research

The most predictable moral argument in support of human cloning is the one commonly used to defend scientific progress in general: The possibility of human cloning stands for an enormous scientific achievement, and achievements as such should always be strengthened and encouraged, and by no means hindered. Of course, technological achievements and scientific advances always come together with potential risks and perils, but technological and scientific development and progress must never be halted, as this would impede evolution and reduce the potential of our species.[201] Cloning is hailed as the so far most illustrious scientific achievement, being the result of the collaboration at the highest possible level between several fields: biology, medicine, genetics, etc. Could we afford such a project to collapse under the weight of objections and fears that we do not even know if they are well-founded? At the end of the day, the ways any scientific achievement will be used is not for scientists to determine; rather, it is the task of politicians and social leaders to decide: Science merely creates possibilities. Irrespective of how the fruits of scientific and technological progress are being used, science must in any case be allowed to develop its full potential. Anything else would only amount to some atavistic revival of Luddism in regard to modern science.[202] The arguments in favor of a right to free scientific research are clearly of ethical nature: They are based upon the moral thesis that science *ought to* be left free to develop its full potential, a view that, while it may also be supported by strong utilitarian arguments, derives its justification primarily from the Kantian tradition.

Immanuel Kant famously classified moral duties on two levels, i.e., as those towards oneself and others, and at the same time – following Grotius', von Puffendorf's and Wolff's train of thought in this – as perfect and imperfect.[203] Kant's classifi-

[201] Ludwig Siep, "Ethical Problems of Stem Cell Research and Stem Cell Transplantation," in *Progress of Science and the Danger of Hubris*, eds. Constantinos Deltas, Eleni Kalokairinou, and Sabine Rogge, 91-99 (Munster: Waxmann, 2006), 93.

[202] Ronald Bailey, "Human Cloning Experiments Should Be Allowed," in *Cloning*, ed. Paul Winters, 73-77 (San Diego, CA: Greenhaven Press, 1998), 74.

[203] Kant, *Groundwork for the Metaphysics of Morals*, 4:421: "I understand by a perfect duty that which permits no exception to the advantage of inclination, and I do have perfect duties that are not merely external but also internal;" see also Kant, *The Metaphysics of Morals*, 6:240, and 6:413; for

cation gives us four possible combinations: [1] perfect duties towards oneself and [2] others, [3] imperfect duties towards oneself and [4] others.

Perfect duties determine certain actions "that must be performed (or, as the case may be, omitted) on every occasion."[204] To suppose otherwise would only lead to a logical contradiction.[205] The moral maxim, for example, that demands that one ought to keep one's promises no matter what, outlines a perfect duty, because any possible alternative maxim, i.e., 'one should never keep one's promises,' or 'one ought to keep one's promises only when one is inclined to do so,' if they became universal laws of nature, would only lead to glaring logical contradictions: The very moment any of these became a universal law, the very idea of promising would just vanish into thin air, and the moral maxim that has just become a universal law would be absolutely meaningless. That is, anyone who is willing to act according to the moral maxims 'one should never keep one's promises,' or 'one should keep

the distinction between perfect and imperfect duties, quite telling is 6:419: "The first principle of duty to oneself lies in the dictum 'live in conformity with nature' (naturae convenienter vive), that is, preserve yourself in the perfection of your nature; the second, in the saying 'make yourself more perfect than mere nature has made you' (perfice te ut finem, perfice te ut medium)."

[204] Jeremy Waldron, "On the Road: Good Samaritans and Compelling Duties," *Santa Clara Law Review* 40, no. 4 (2000): 1071.

[205] See Kant, *Groundwork for the Metaphysics of Morals*, 4:424: "One must be able to will that a maxim of our action should become a universal law: this is the canon of the moral judgment of this action in general. Some actions are so constituted that their maxim cannot even be thought without contradiction as a universal law of nature, much less could one will that it ought to become one." For an excellent analysis on duties to oneself and to others, and in particular on perfect and imperfect duties to oneself, see Thomas E. Hill, *The Blackwell Guide to Kant's Ethics* (Malden: John Wiley & Sons, 2009), 229ff.

one's promises only when one is willing to do so,' would have already deprived herself of the possibility of following either of these maxims and breaking her promises, since in that case no one would have any reason to make promises anymore, knowing in advance that everybody else endorses one of these maxims. Inherent in the very concept of promising is the moral obligation to keep promises, just as inherent the very concept of property is the moral obligation to respect property. Anything else is logically impossible.

Noncompliance with imperfect duties, on the other hand, leads to no logical contradiction, and this is why imperfect duties "bind us in a much looser way, leaving ample room for personal discretion."[206] That being said, we are by our nature inclined to favor actions that are commonly regarded as instances of imperfect duties, while rejecting actions that contradict the maxims that give rise to those duties: In short, even if these duties are not strict and any maxim that suggests we should not obey them would not be self-defeating, it is natural for us to *will* these duties to be observed, and this is what makes complying with these duties morally preferably.[207] Kant cites the cultivation of one's talents as an example of imperfect moral duties towards oneself. One who, for whatever reason, fails in the cultivation of a particular talent – or simply neglects it – is not morally reprehensible for doing so. Moreover, any moral maxim that would justify not developing or neglecting one's talents might well hold as a universal law of nature; there would be no logical contradiction in such a maxim: We can imagine a world in which no one would bother to develop any potential. However, none would be expected to

[206] Daniel Statman, "Who Needs Imperfect Duties?" *American Philosophical Quarterly* 33, no. 2 (1996): 211.
[207] Michael Stocker, "Acts, Perfect Duties, and Imperfect Duties," *The Review of Metaphysics* 20, no. 3 (1967): 507.

will such a maxim to be elevated to the status of a universal law of nature. To put it in Kant's words:

> [...] although a nature could still subsist in accordance with such a universal law, though then the human being (like the South Sea Islanders) would think only of letting his talents rust and applying his life merely to idleness, amusement, procreation, in a word, to enjoyment; yet it is impossible for him to will that this should become a universal law of nature, or that it should be implanted in us as such by natural instinct. For as a rational being he necessarily wills that all the faculties in him should be developed, because they are serviceable and given to him for all kinds of possible aims.[208]

Kant's line of thought presents an extremely strong line of defense for the view that science should be allowed to flourish, to develop to its full potential unimpeded. For one thing, it is an imperfect duty for geneticists, just as it is for every other rational being, to strive for the development of 'all the faculties in them' as innate, inalienable properties of their nature; moreover, the development of these faculties would be 'serviceable to all for all kinds of possible aims,' hence it would be 'impossible' for anyone *to will* that any alternative maxim would become a universal law of nature: While a nature could still subsist if our societies remained technologically and scientifically undeveloped, any maxim that would support free and unfettered research, and favor technological and scientific progress, would make life much easier, more creative, and

---

[208] Kant, *Groundwork for the Metaphysics of Morals*, 4:423.

generally more worth-living, so it would be against our nature to will otherwise: It is only reasonable to will that such a maxim, and not some alternative, would be elevated to the status of a universal law of nature. In short, the unfettered progress of science could be seen as an imperfect duty for moral agents; and if this also includes the unfettered development of human reproductive cloning, then so be it.

In support of the above, today states such as Germany,[209] Italy[210] and Slovenia[211] explicitly mention that freedom of scientific research enjoys constitutional protection,[212] while in several other countries, such as Canada and the United States, freedom of scientific research is protected as an essential component of freedom of thought and expression; in the United States, in particular, freedom of scientific research is usually considered to be protected by the First Amendment, which protects freedom of speech. The 13th Article of the *Charter of Fundamental Rights of the European Union* states that "The arts and scientific research shall be free of constraint. Academic freedom shall be respected."[213] The explanation of this

---

[209] Grundgesetz für die Bundesrepublik Deutschland, *Bundesanzeiger* I, 968, article 5, §3: "Arts and sciences, research and teaching shall be free. The freedom of teaching shall not release any person from allegiance to the constitution."

[210] Costituzione della Repubblica Italiana, *Gazzetta Ufficiale* 298, article 33: "The Republic guarantees the freedom of the arts and sciences, which may be freely taught."

[211] Ustava Republike Slovenije, *Uradni list Republike Slovenije*, no. 33/91-I, 42/97, 66/2000, 24/03, 69/04, 68/06, 47/13 and 75/16, article 59: "The freedom of scientific and artistic endeavour shall be guaranteed."

[212] See Amedeo Santosuosso, "Freedom of Research and Constitutional Law: Some Critical Points," in *An Anthology on Freedom of Scientific Research*, eds. Simona Giordano, John Coggon, and Marco Cappato, 73-82 (London, and New York: Bloomsbury, 2014).

[213] European Commission, *EU Charter of Fundamental Rights*, 2000, https://

article, as it appears in the Official Journal of the European Union, makes it clear that,

> This right is deduced primarily from the right to freedom of thought and expression. It is to be exercised having regard to Article 1 [which demands respect for human dignity] and may be subject to the limitations authorized by Article 10 [that regards freedom of thought, conscience and religion] of the ECHR.[214]

Against this background, freedom of scientific research is often considered not only as a right that should be granted to researchers alone, but also as "the human right to enjoy the benefits of scientific progress and its applications,"[215] and this means that its protection should be an obligation of the state, especially because free "scientific expression – considering its importance to the discovery and dissemination of certain truths about the world – contains sufficient social value,"[216] while science free from calculations of social utility and political expediency best serves the state and society. It almost goes without saying that the freedom of scientific research is not limited to the phase of selecting research objectives, instruments, and methods, but *also* concerns *the application of*

---

commission.europa.eu/aid-development-cooperation-fundamental-rights/your-rights-eu/eu-charter-fundamental-rights_en.

[214] *Official Journal of the European Union*, C 303/17 – 14.12.2007.

[215] Audrey Chapman, and Jessica Wyndham, "A Human Right to Science," *Science* 340, no. 6138 (2013): 1291. See also, Alf Butenschøn Skre, and Asbjørn Eide, "The Human Right to Benefit from Advances in Science and Promotion of Openly Accessible Publications," *Nordic Journal of Human Rights* 31, no. 3 (2013): 427-453.

[216] Santosuosso, 76.

scientific results insofar as this would further advance scientific research.

This reasoning seems to be effective, but, in my opinion, not to the extent – nor in the direction – that those who invoke it believe it is. It may indeed be the case that the freedom of scientific research should be regarded as an imperfect (or broad) moral duty. However, this does not mean that research should be absolutely free in all cases and regardless of other morally relevant parameters: As it is with imperfect duties, this one is also subject to limitations and constraints that often arise from other duties that conflict with it. Our imperfect duty to love our neighbors, for example, may be constrained at some point by our duty to love our parents.[217] Similarly, the scientist's duty to develop her skills and expertise to its potential may also be limited by some other duty, that may seem equally compelling and binding, for example the duty to maintain social order, or to defend human dignity.[218] In other words, although the freedom of scientific research *as such* stands as a duty, it may be that *in a given situation* scientists and researchers should, in their best moral judgement, give priority to another duty over this one.

And even if we assume some sort of moral imperative regarding the unfettered development of science and research, it does not necessarily follow that there is also an imperative

---

[217] Kant, *The Metaphysics of Morals*, 6:390.

[218] The defense of human dignity is the reason for invoking Article 11 of the UNESCO Universal Declaration on the Human Genome and Human Rights of 11th November 1997: "modes of practice contrary to human dignity, such as the cloning of human beings for reproductive purposes, are not permitted." Reproductive human cloning is further prohibited by the First Additional Protocol of 18th February 1998 to the Council of Europe Convention on Human Rights and Biomedicine of 4th April 1997, and Article 3, §2 of the Charter of Fundamental Rights of the European Union of December 7, 2000.

to accept, implement and exploit every possible outcome. It sounds plausible that scientists have a moral obligation to constantly explore all possibilities in order to advance knowledge, map still unexplored territories and conquer ever more distant horizons. In this regard, it would be morally unjustifiable to impede research related to reproductive cloning, even if it involved the cloning of human beings: This would indeed be at odds with the imperfect duty to expand our capabilities and enhance our potential as individuals and species. But the *way in which* research on reproductive cloning should be conducted, the directions in which it should go, *whether* it should lead to the actual cloning of human beings, or be stopped at an earlier stage as is the case at present, *when* and *under what conditions* reproductive cloning should be applied to human beings, none of this is at all relevant to the *general* duty to advance scientific knowledge; on the contrary, all these are moral questions in their own right, aimed at exploring the moral distance between what is *achievable* or *possible*, and what is *proper* or *right*. And if the former is to be preserved and promoted, the latter is to be debated by bioethics. Pure scientific research, as several ethicists aptly note, must pursue what is *achievable* and be indifferent to the question of whether something is *right*. As Bernard Rollin puts it, "science is value-free; hence ethics-free, and thus it is society's job (if anyone's) to articulate the ethical implications of science and technology."[219]

Of course, one could argue that human reproductive cloning is probably a *sine qua non* for science and technology in the field of reproductive cloning to develop as far as possible[220] – as well as all related fields: Even the most thorough and well-doc-

---

[219] Rollin, 53.

[220] Carmel Shalev, "Human Cloning and Human Rights: A Commentary," *Health and Human Rights* 6, no. 1 (2002): 139: "Major advances in science have historically been unforeseen and surprising: we look for one thing and

umented theoretical model should be tested in real life in order to be perfected. I believe that this is not true. And even if it were, it does not follow that human reproductive cloning should be allowed in all cases. As for my first contention, I will rely on two arguments that I believe are similar. First, consider scientific research in the field of nuclear physics, especially nuclear fission, and its potential uses: It led to the construction of nuclear weapons, on the one hand, and to nuclear energy as a natural resource for mankind, on the other. Could it be argued that the only way to study the effects of nuclear fission and perfect the scientific knowledge associated with it – to ultimately make nuclear energy useful for peaceful purposes – was to drop an atomic bomb on Hiroshima and Nagasaki? As developments in the field show, such an assertion would be false, for nuclear physics has since made great strides without the need to drop a similar bomb elsewhere, and although, by the way, nuclear testing in nature has also been banned. But even if there were no other possibility of scientific progress, would this justify the monstrous humanitarian catastrophe caused by the dropping of the bomb? To answer this question in the affirmative would be to overlook the nature of science and technology, which outlines both their ends and their means – and at the same time sets limits to them: Science and technology do not exist for their own sake, but only as tools for improving human living conditions. It would be completely nonsensical to pursue and strive for science and technology in a way that only harms humans or even destroys the entire species – because, next to anything else, there is actually no need for this: Although some are indeed shorter and easier to take, there is not only one path that leads to scientific development. I can think of no better proof for this than the infamous 'children of Willowbrook' case.

---

find by chance something else far more significant."

From 1956 to 1971 Saul Krugman, the director of Willowbrook Psychiatric Hospital on Staten Island, conducted experimental research to isolate and study the hepatitis virus. Krugman had reason to believe that G-globulin could induce lasting immunity to the virus, but he needed to test his theory on living subjects. To that end he decided to use inmates, intellectually disabled minors who were not carriers of the virus: He intentionally infected healthy children with the virus, and then administered globulin to some of them. His experiments confirmed his initial suspicions about the effectiveness of G-globulin in producing immunity to the virus. He also demonstrated that infectious hepatitis (type A), transmitted via the fecal-oral route, and the more serious 'serum' hepatitis (type B), transmitted via blood, bodily secretions, and sexual contact, are caused by two immunologically distinct viruses, and that only the second can be fatal.[221] Krugman's studies were instrumental in developing scientific knowledge and treatment for the hepatitis virus, saving the lives of millions; at the same time, however, they represent "the most unethical medical experiments ever performed on children in the United States."[222] Around the same time Baruch Bloomberg managed to isolate the hepatitis B virus strain in his laboratory, and came to the same conclusions as Krugman, but without using humans as guinea pigs. This probably explains why Bloomberg was awarded the Nobel Prize in 1976 for his contributions to physiology and medicine, while Krugman became the central figure in a heated debate about the ethical parameters that should (or should not) apply to scientific research.[223]

---

[221] See Robert Ward, Saul Krugman, Joan P. Giles, A. Milton Jacobs, and Oscar Bodansky, "Infectious Hepatitis: Studies of Its Natural History and Prevention," *New England Journal of Medicine* 258, no. 9 (1958): 407-416.

[222] Paul A. Offit, *Vaccinated* (New York: Harper Collins, 2007), 27.

[223] See, for example, Henry Beecher, "Ethics and Clinical Research," *New*

Of course, these two analogical arguments I have used to support my view are not conclusive. After all, analogical reasoning can only demonstrate and provide good evidence, but cannot lead to conclusions that follow from logical necessity: Both the case of the atomic bomb and the case of the children of Willowbrook may be similar, but they are by no means identical to reproductive cloning. In my opinion, the extent of the similarities between these cases is sufficient to conclude that genetics could make progress without the need for actual human cloning. I am aware that it could be argued against my view that the application of reproductive cloning to humans, should it ever occur, will in no way entail the catastrophic consequences of a nuclear explosion or be marked by the moral failures of Krugman's experiments. In making these arguments, then, I have sought to show, first, that scientific progress never goes in only one direction, and second, that not all paths it may take are equally consistent with its true nature and mission. In short, I believe that reproductive cloning and all related sciences could still develop to their full potential and even reach the level of perfection required for successful human cloning without having to move to the stage of actually cloning humans for that purpose. Thus, the argument that the legitimate pursuit of scientific progress in cloning requires the cloning of humans is, in my view, neither unassailable nor does it have the probative force that those who invoke it believe it to have.

II. Begetting biologically related offspring

It is clear that human cloning is primarily intended as a means of procreation, which could be an *alternative* for many people.

England Journal of Medicine 274, no. 24 (1966): 1354-1360. For a broader contemporary critical consideration of the Willowbrook experiment and the limits of scientific research, see Tom Regan, "Empty Cages: Animal Rights and Vivisection," in *Animal Ethics: Past and Present Perspectives*, ed. Evangelos Protopapadakis, 179-196 (Berlin: Logos Verlag, 2012), 184-186.

For some people, however, cloning would be the only way to produce offspring – if, of course, were legalized. This is especially true for infertile couples: For them, cloning would be the only way to have biologically related children, because somatic cell cloning does not depend on genetic material from reproductive cells. Instead, genetic material can be taken from the somatic cells of one or both future parents (in the future it will probably be possible to recombine genetic material from the somatic cells of both parents),[224] then inserted into an enucleated egg cell of a donor, and finally implanted into the uterus of the future mother, or even a surrogate mother.

Cloning also seems to be the only solution for couples who are fertile, but where one or both individuals either suffer from a serious hereditary disease or have a genetic predisposition that makes natural reproduction unwise. In this case, the woman provides the egg. The nucleus is then replaced either by a nucleus from her partner's somatic cells – if she is the carrier of the disease or the undesirable genetic predisposition, or by a nucleus from her own somatic cells – if her partner is the carrier. In either case, the resulting embryo will be free of the disease or unwanted genetic predisposition, and this makes cloning in such cases a prospective therapeutic practice and a public health option. Moreover, we can assume that the genes responsible for inherited diseases would inevitably disappear from the gene pool of our species in the long run if cloning were applied on a large scale to carriers of inherited diseases. On the one hand, this would be a prime example of procreative beneficence, i.e., the production of offspring with the best chance of living as unencumbered a life as possible, and on the other hand, the resources that have so far been wast-

---

[224] See Carson Strong, "Reproductive Cloning Combined with Genetic Modification," *Journal of Medical Ethics* 31 (2005): 654-658, esp. 655.

ed on the treatment of hereditary diseases such as sickle cell anemia, Huntington's disease or hemophilia could be used for the treatment of other, non-genetic – and thus not in advance preventable – diseases such as cancer, Alzheimer's disease and AIDS. In the eyes of several ethicists, mostly utilitarians, both eliminating preventable disease in our offspring and maximizing resources to minimize pain seem to be the only morally defensible options.

Moreover, it can also be argued that cloning provides a reproductive opportunity for people who do not fall into the usual pattern of genetic mating – or, any mating at all – i.e., same-sex couples,[225] as well as single people who desire biologically related children. I know that the debate over human reproductive cloning in such cases is for some like trying to run before you can walk: There is still a strong moral controversy over whether same-sex couples or single parents should adopt children at all, fueling a heated debate. As one would expect, this debate more often than not mixes scientific evidence with religious or metaphysical beliefs, personal attitudes, and so on, sometimes resulting in far more heated controversy than any other typical ethical debate would allow. In this regard, I will take a neutral position, even more so since my discussion of human reproductive cloning as a means of exercising the right to reproductive freedom does not really require me to take sides. Instead, in what follows I will equate same-sex couples and single people with infertile couples and couples who carry genetically transmitted diseases or undesirable genetic predispositions. I believe that there are good reasons for this: a) *there are already* same-sex couples who sometimes want offspring who are biologically related either to both of them, or at least to one of

---

[225] See, for example, David Orentliche, "Beyond Cloning: Expanding Reproductive Options for Same-sex Couples," *Brooklyn Law Review* 66, no. 3 (2001): 653.

them,[226] while there are also already several legal frameworks that allow same-sex couples to adopt, b) *there are already* single-parent families (either because one parent has died, or the parents are divorced and one of them is absent, etc.), while there are already several legal frameworks that allow adoption for single parents; c) in the event that human reproductive cloning ever becomes a legitimate reproductive option, same-sex couples as well as single parents will make use of it for exactly the same reasons that a typical infertile couple – or a couple for whom natural reproduction is out of the question for the reasons previously mentioned – would today, namely, only because they are unable to have offspring that are biologically related to them in some other way.[227] For these reasons, I have chosen to discuss the right to reproductive freedom with respect to these three categories of potential parents as if they were a single category, even though I know that they differ greatly in all other respects: For what is morally significant for our discussion in all three cases is nothing other than the fact that these people are unable to have offspring biologically related to them in ways other than reproductive cloning.

If legitimizing human reproductive cloning is the only way for people who fall into these categories to produce offspring, then banning cloning would seems to directly affect these people[228]

---

[226] The possibility of adoption – despite its undisputed moral value – in no way replaces the possibility of having biologically related offspring. This is, by the way, also the reason why in the vast majority of cases adoption is chosen when the possibility of having a biological offspring is no longer given. See Mary Warnock, *Is There a Right to Have Children?* (Oxford: Oxford University Press, 2002), 40.

[227] Ahlberg, and Brighouse, 552.

[228] John A. Robertson, "The Question of Human Cloning," *Hastings Center Report* 24, no. 2 (1194): 13: "[...] the right of married and arguably even unmarried persons to procreate is a fundamental constitutional right that cannot be restricted unless clearly necessary to protect compelling state interests."

and interfere with their right to reproductive freedom,[229] which is sometimes considered a human right, and sometimes *merely* a moral right.[230] Human rights are generally considered to be privileges that every human being is entitled to *only by virtue of his or her nature*, i.e. only because they belong to the species *Homo sapiens*.[231] All human beings, for example, precisely because they are human beings, and without having to fulfill any other condition, i.e., regardless of their sex or gender, nationality, physical or intellectual abilities, and so on, are recognized as having the right to freely express their views, to practice their chosen religion, to fulfill their religious duties, etc. Moral rights, on the other hand, are 'time-slice' cultural institutions: They are the result of an ineffable agreement, a covenant between moral agents within a particular historical and social context. In other words, the much-discussed moral right to die (or, rather, to be allowed to choose the time and circumstances or manner of one's own death), which is central to the euthanasia debate, is meaningful only in the context of a moral community that accepts the validity of this right and grants it to its members. Moral agents can invoke this right and make claims based on it only in the context of a particular moral community, on the basis of a preexisting moral convention that makes the invocation of this right meaningful, but in no case by invoking their human nature in general. This right might be not only unacceptable,

---

[229] Lynn Freedman, and Stephen Isaacs, "Human Rights and Reproductive Choice," *Studies in Family Planning* 24, no. 1 (1993): 18-30, esp. 20-21.

[230] On the nature of human rights as claim-rights, liberty-rights, power-rights, or immunity-rights, as well as on their relation to moral rights, see Carl Wellman, "The Nature of International Human Rights," in *The Moral Dimensions of Human Rights*, ed. Carl Wellman, 71-84 (Oxford: Oxford University Press, 2011).

[231] James Griffin, "First Steps in an Account of Human Rights," *European Journal of Philosophy* 9, no. 3 (2001): 306.

but also completely incomprehensible in a different historical or social context. For example, while the right to vigilante justice is unacceptable – even incomprehensible – in the Western world today, it has not always been so, while in certain cultural settings this right is still considered more central than other commonly accepted rights. Human rights, on the contrary, are seen as atemporal, timeless normative principles that govern relations between individuals, or their interaction with the state.[232] It follows that they are granted a much broader frame of reference and a much broader scope of application – since they derive from general human nature and a supposedly *universal* morality, no matter how strongly this view is contested, and the very concept of human rights is questioned.[233] Against this background, I will discuss whether and how the right to reproductive freedom could be related to human reproductive cloning, whether it is seen as a purely moral right, or as a human right.

In its first aspect, that of a fundamental human right, the right to reproductive freedom was outlined at the International Conference on Human Rights held in Tehran in 1968: "Parents have a basic human right to determine freely and responsibly the number and the spacing of their children."[234] The wording of the final resolution of the UN Third World Population Conference held in Bucharest in 1974, seems to

---

[232] John Rawls, *The Law of Peoples* (Cambridge, MA: Harvard University Press, 1999), 80-83.

[233] See, for example, James H. Hutson, "The Bill of Rights and the American Revolutionary Experience," in *A Culture of Rights*, eds. Michael J. Lacey, and Knud Haakonssen, 62-97 (Cambridge: Cambridge University Press, 1991), 67: "[...] the public's penchant for asserting its rights outran its ability to analyze them and to reach a consensus about their scope and meaning."

[234] United Nations, "Proclamation of Teheran," in *Final Act of the International Conference on Human Rights* (New York: United Nations, 1968), article 16, A/Conf. 32/41.

broaden the scope by referring not only to couples, but also to individuals:

> All couples and individuals have the basic right to decide freely and responsibly the number and spacing of their children and to have the information, education and means to do so; the responsibility of couples and individuals in the exercise of this right takes into account the needs of their living and future children – and their responsibilities towards the community.[235]

The most striking difference here is that the term 'parents' was omitted and replaced instead by the phrase 'couples and individuals.' In a later related judgment, the right to reproductive freedom was defined as follows:

> Every couple and every individual has the right to decide freely and responsibly whether or not to have children as well as to determine their number and spacing, and to have information, education and means to do so.[236]

This last definition makes the right to reproductive freedom seem much more nuanced: According to this new phrasing, this right includes both the right *not to procreate*, possibly through the use of various contraceptive methods or through abortion, and the right to reproduce. The second aspect, the

---

[235] United Nations, *Report of the United Nations World Population Conference* (New York: United Nations, 1975), II, §7.

[236] United Nations, *Report of the World Conference of the International Woman's Year* (New York: United Nations, 1976), E/Conf. 66/34, I, §12.

right to reproduce, is considered by many[237] to also imply a right *to choose the means by which* it is to be exercised, including all modern technological options available, such as *in vitro* fertilization, ovarian donation, surrogacy, etc. The use of assisted reproduction techniques, such as those mentioned above, can be considered part of the right to reproductive freedom, as the state is obliged to:

> Make available to individuals and couples through an institutionalized system, such as a national family planning programme, such information, service and means as will enable them to determine freely the number of their children and the intervals at which they will have them.[238]

Given the above and the fact that cloning is a *service* that allows individuals and couples to decide freely, i.e., according to their own free will – unhindered by natural heteronomy – whether and how many children they want to have, human reproductive cloning should be available not only to those for whom it is the only way to have biologically related children, but also to all who would consider it as one option among several others.[239] In other words, just as any woman, even if she is absolutely capable of conceiving and carrying her own child, is entitled to choose in vitro fertilization treatment and subsequently have her fetus

---

[237] Dan Brock, "Cloning Human Beings: An Assessment of the Ethical Issues Pro and Con," in *Clones and Clones: Facts and Fantasies about Human Cloning*, eds. Martha Nussbaum, and Cass R. Sunstein, 141-164 (New York: W. W. Norton Co., 1999).

[238] United Nations, *Report of the World Conference of the International Woman's Year*, IV, §2.

[239] Helga Kuhse, "Should Cloning Be Banned for the Sake of the Child?" *Poiesis and Praxis* 1 (2001): 28.

carried by a surrogate mother, so too should cloning be available to any fertile and healthy heterosexual couple as a reproductive option, even if they could have children either through physical or in vitro fertilization. According to the UN report I cited above, it is the duty of the state to provide all available and legitimate means and services to couples and individuals. That is, unless there are indeed good reasons that human reproductive cloning either should not be considered as a reproductive service and means, or should be excluded from this duty of the state.

The validity and weight of the above argument is, of course, greatly enhanced in the case of persons for whom cloning is the only means of begetting children: If other options were also available besides cloning, then a ban on human reproductive cloning would simply be an interference with the right *to choose* between different means, i.e., a limitation of the scope of that right. However, if no other option is available, then it is the right to reproductive freedom in general that is compromised, and not any particular aspect of it. In sum, to ban human reproductive cloning is to deny some people the right to reproduce, and everyone else the right to decide for themselves the appropriate means to do so. In light of this, preventing scientific research into human reproductive cloning means either partial or complete violation of the right to procreate. As Dan Brock notes,

> The reproductive right relevant to human cloning is a negative right, that is, a right to use assisted reproductive technologies without interference by the government or others when made available by a willing provider. The choice of an assisted means of reproduction, such as surrogacy, can be defended as included within reproduc-

tive freedom, even when it is not the only means
for individuals to reproduce, just as the choice
among different means of preventing conception
is protected by reproductive freedom.[240]

At this point it should be noted that the right to reproductive
freedom, like all rights of the type: 'Every human should have
a right to X, just because she is a human being,' should be understood as overriding any possible restriction, necessity, or
adverse inclination. This means that non-compliance with the
right to reproductive freedom is always morally unjustifiable,
regardless of how burdensome or undesirable compliance
with that right would be: If every human being should have
a right to something, the only way to prove that one does not
have the right to something is to show that one is not human;
everything else should be morally irrelevant. Consider the
case of China a few decades ago, when couples were forbidden
to have more than two children: No matter how documented
or socially justified such a ban might have been, it would still
be morally unjustifiable if reproductive freedom is indeed a
human right. Human rights are never subject to contingency
or feasibility. To put it in the words of John Stuart Mill,

> if all mankind minus one, were of one opinion,
> and only one person were of the contrary opin-
> ion, mankind would be no more justified in si-
> lencing that one person, than he, if he had the
> power, would be justified in silencing mankind.[241]

---

[240] Brock, 144.

[241] John Stuart Mill, *On Liberty: Utilitarianism and Other Essays*, eds. Mark
Philip, and Frederick Rosen (Oxford: Oxford University Press, 2015), 19.

Ronald Dworkin seems to follow in Mill's footsteps on this issue. In his view, rights take precedence over everything else in
cases of conflict: It is as if they confer on their holders a kind
of *absolute advantage*, by virtue of which persons are entitled
to be acted upon or allowed to act in certain ways, even when
the common good is at stake, or it would be better served if
they were treated differently.[242] In a word, according to Dworkin, *rights trump utility*. Against this background, then, a ban
on human reproductive cloning would in any case mean – irrespective of the reasons that have led to it – an unjustifiable
violation of a right, either the right to procreate in general, or
the right to choose the means one thinks appropriate or convenient.[243] According to this line of reasoning, it always boils
down to the fact that human reproductive cloning should be
allowed either as an alternative, or as the only way out to have
biologically related offspring, so that the right to reproductive
freedom is not violated.

The above argument seems strong, but one cannot help
pointing out some weaknesses. These weaknesses, it must be
emphasized at the outset, do not show that human reproductive should generally remain forbidden, but just that allowing
it cannot be adequately grounded in the right to reproductive
freedom. First, human reproductive cloning today is only a
probability, and by no means a *possibility*. For, unlike the cloning of sheep or frogs, the point of human cloning, at least according to the Kantian view[244] – and so far no other view has

---

[242] Ronald Dworkin, "Rights as Trumps," in *Theories of Rights*, ed. J. Waldron,
153-167 (Oxford: Oxford University Press, 1984); see also his *Taking Rights
Seriously* (New York: Harvard University Press, 1978), 364ff.

[243] Carson Strong, "Cloning and Infertility," *Cambridge Quarterly of
Healthcare Ethics* 7 (1998): 279-293, n. 1.

[244] This is the second formulation of Kant's categorical imperative: "Act so
that you use humanity, as much in your own person as in the person of

been openly advocated – is not to create a new human being, the clone of an existing or once-existing human being, merely for experimental purposes; rather, human reproductive cloning aims to create human beings who will have the same prospects as any other human being; in other words, cloning promises to create human beings who will be capable of leading lives as *worth living* as any other human being,[245] i.e., human beings who will have normal life expectancy, the same prospects for quality of life, etc. If the purpose were any other, e.g., the advancement of scientific knowledge or the perfection of cloning, then the clone would be nothing more than a *mere means to an end* that would be absolutely alien to the clone and outside the very clone's will, an end to which the clone was never given the chance to consent, and which we have good reason to assume would never receive the clone's consent. Aside from the fact that this contradicts the famous second formulation of Kant's categorical imperative, which for some should be the cornerstone of medical and research ethics (when it comes to research on humans), it sends shivers down the spine to think that Joseph Mengele, the infamous *angel of death* at the Auschwitz death camp, thought of and treated his inmates in exactly this way.[246] Lest Mengele's spirit be revived, human reproductive cloning could only be an issue if the dignity, autonomy and best interests of the clone are protected. Science, however, is currently far from being able to provide a guarantee of this.

---

every other, always at the same time as end and never merely as means." It is worth noting that this axiom according to Kant is not empirical, but derives from pure reason, because on the one hand it is universal, and on the other hand it is not posited as a subjective end, but as an objective one. See Kant, *Groundwork for the Metaphysics of Morals*, 4:429; cf. 4:436.

[245] Ahlberg, and Brighouse, 540.

[246] See, inter alia, Vivien Spitz, *Doctors from Hell: The Horrific Account of Nazi Experiments on Humans* (New York: Scientific Publications, 2005).

Of course, if the only issue were lack of guarantees, one could argue that cloning is not significantly different from other methods of reproduction, including natural reproduction: In none of these methods is there any guarantee that the resulting human being will live a life worth living, at least insofar as a life worth living depends on her genetically inherited phenotype and genotype: Genetic abnormalities, congenital disorders, unforeseen complications at birth, however rare, are always likely. In the case of human cloning, however, such failures would not only be a low probability, but as things stand today, serious genetic complications would be certain: If geneticists today decided to proceed with human cloning, they would rightly have to fear, not just expect, that the clone produced would struggle with respiratory and circulatory problems, would age prematurely, etc., because that is how mammalian cloning has worked so far. It appears that the science and technology required for risk-free cloning is not yet available, or perhaps there are inherent weaknesses in the overall concept of cloning organisms as advanced and sophisticated as mammals.[247] This means that – again, given the current state of affairs regarding the possibilities and weaknesses of cloning – if clones were to be created in the near future, it would not be for the purpose of creating new human beings that could potentially live a life worth-living, but for the purpose of achieving some other end that would be alien to the clones themselves. Thus, it could reasonably be argued that this would violate the created clone's right to a satisfying human life on the one hand,[248] but more importantly, that in the face of the clone humanity would not have been treated simultaneously as an end, but only as a means. And while it

---

[247] Dan Brock, "Cloning Human Beings."
[248] Strong, "Cloning and Infertility," 280.

remains doubtful and controversial whether it is morally justifiable to bring into existence human beings with less than minimal chance of a decent life, it is really difficult to challenge the view that humans should always be treated also as ends in themselves.

The conflict would be settled only if we could consider the clone merely as a means of satisfying its progenitors' right to reproductive freedom and disregard the question of whether the clone has any right at all, especially the right to a life worth living. This would, however, be a significant paradigm shift with respect to human reproduction, in which the resulting children are often indeed a means to certain ends of their progenitors (to be safe, to entertain the fear of death by the sense of continued life through their offspring, to satisfy practical needs, etc.), but they are nonetheless valuable as ends in their own right. This means, though, that we would have to recognize two categories of biological offspring: [a] non-clones, who would be born to live as worth-living a life as possible, and who would be both means to alien purposes and ends in themselves at the same time, and [b] clones, who would be born to live a life we would in advance be sure that it will be not worth-living – or, at least, not as much worth-living as that of non-clones – who would be created only as a means to an end, be it the exercise of their progenitors' right to reproductive freedom, or scientific progress and the advancement of cloning technology, or anything else. If so, respecting the right to reproductive freedom would mean disrespecting human dignity in the face of clones, assuming that clones will be human beings in the full. Against this background, the right to reproductive freedom cannot be unconditional like, say, the right to life, but it should be limited either by the duty to protect an even more fundamental right, namely the right of the clone to live a reasonably decent life, or by respect for human dignity, which would be compromised in the face of clones who would be treated as second-class, lesser human beings. This must be true *even if* for some individuals or couples human reproductive cloning is indeed the only hope for begetting offspring, since: [a] the resulting clones would be treated as *quasi persons* from the outset – at least in comparison with non-clones, since their creation would be intended from the outset solely to serve some end alien to them; [b] the procreation of offspring by cloning would condemn them, as things stand today, to a life much more arduous and limited than that of naturally conceived offspring, and [c] it would mean accepting *de facto* the view that human beings could sometimes be regarded only as means to alien ends. Given the above, and the fact that the scientific evidence available today clearly shows the limitations and weaknesses of cloning, which ensure that the clones produced would have a poor quality of life and a low life expectancy,[249] it could be argued that human reproductive cloning cannot be considered part of the right to reproductive freedom: As things now stand, cloning is not yet a legitimate reproductive option like, say, surrogacy or in vitro fertilization,[250] so banning it doesn't affect the right to reproductive freedom.

From a very different, a utilitarian perspective, it could be argued that not allowing human reproductive cloning as a legitimate reproductive option would impede scientific progress in this area in the same way that not allowing in vitro fertilization as a reproductive alternative would have done: Any effects of this technique on the health of the clone could not be assessed in terms of their magnitude, scope, and significance

---

[249] National Bioethics Advisory Commission, *Cloning Human Beings: Report and Recommendations of the National Bioethics Advisory Commission* (Rockville, MD: National Bioethics Advisory Commission, 1997), 34.
[250] Ibid., 64-65.

until at least one human clone had been produced. Opponents of this view argue that even in the event that the creation of a single human clone were sufficient to perfect cloning (which is utterly unrealistic), this would still be morally reprehensible because that first clone would have been used merely as a means to an end. But then the rigid attitude of not using humans merely as a means to an end seems devastating to scientific progress. If this view prevailed, there would be little progress in science: Marie and Pierre Curie would never have discovered the effects of radium hadn't they treated humanity in their faces merely as a means to an end by exposing themselves to the forces of radiation in self-experimentation; the same is true of Jonas Silk, who tested his polio vaccine on himself and his family, and of some other researchers who regarded themselves only as a means to an end in order to advance their science: *Mutatis mutandis*, every time a drug, substance, or technology must be tested for the first time on even a single human being, the human being in question is, in fact, treated only as a means.[251] But if this were not the case, kidney or heart transplants would never have been available, nor would the life-saving effects of insulin or penicillin. By analogy, it is also inappropriate to base the moral debate over human reproductive cloning solely on the intrinsic, absolute value of human beings.[252] If the potential benefits to humanity outweigh the possible dangers, any risk can be morally justified.

I must confess that I remain skeptical of the arguments for human reproductive cloning. In addition to the considerations I made in the previous section when discussing free-

[251] John A. Robertson, "A Ban on Cloning and Cloning Research is Unjustified," *Testimony Presented to the National Bioethics Advisory Commission*, March 14, 1997.

[252] National Bioethics Advisory Commission, 65.

dom of research and scientific freedom in general, I also be-lieve that: [a] The analogy between cloning and other scientif-ic achievements, e.g., heart transplantation, is not very strong. For example, the first heart transplant operations – either successful or unsuccessful – thanks to which our knowledge in this field has been perfected so that today these operations are characterized by a very high success rate and the lives of millions of people are saved, were performed on patients who had given their consent freely and in full awareness of the pos-sibilities, which cannot be expected of the first clones in any way, since it is impossible that they consented to their creation in advance. [b] In all previous scientific advances, the risk was merely incidental and based mainly on ignorance of how the human body would respond to techniques that had already been used with high success rates in animals. In the case of cloning, however, this is not true: Cloning has not yet been applied with high success rates in other species, while in all cases it has resulted to serious issues for the clone.[253] But more importantly, [c] performing a risky heart transplant for the first time on a human being who would be doomed anyway is quite different from making a clone that has no chance of a life worth living and would never have come into existence without our interference; the former has a good chance of increasing overall happiness in the world if the operation is successful, and there is no chance that it will decrease happi-ness in any other case, since the person in question is doomed

---

[253] Rollin, 62: "To attempt cloning today, via the technology that produced Dolly, would clearly violate established medical-ethical principles, since hundreds of attempts would be required, and risk of late term spontaneous abortion threatening the life of the mother would be significant. Furthermore, we are not yet in a position to judge the potential deleterious consequences to the cloned child, and thus, again, it would be immoral to proceed with cloning in a cavalier fashion."

anyway, while the latter will definitely not increase overall happiness (assuming we know that the clone will not live a life worth living), and it is certain to increase overall pain.

Another strong objection to the relevance of the right to reproductive freedom as an argument that supports human reproductive cloning is that this right does not seem to operate in the case of cloning as it does with other methods of assisted reproduction. To illustrate this, let us examine the following thought experiment. Suppose an infertile couple decides to undergo in vitro fertilization and implant the fertilized egg into a surrogate mother who has voluntarily and selflessly agreed to assist in this endeavor. However, the current legal framework in the country where the couple lives has not had time to adapt to new developments in artificial insemination, and therefore neither in vitro fertilization nor the use of a surrogate mother is allowed. The couple in our example could invoke their moral right to procreate, the exercise of which is prevented by the current legal framework, and consequently turn to a supreme state, transnational, or international court to enforce it. Another couple in the same position in a society where both in vitro fertilization and the use of a surrogate mother are permitted might weight the merits of the case and ultimately decide not to exercise their right to procreate, either by relinquishing it or by reserving the right to exercise it in the future. However, the same does not seem to apply to human reproductive cloning. Today, no one can expect to exercise their right to reproduce by cloning, at least not in the near future. One can only hope that in the future it may be possible to exercise this right using cloning as an assisted reproduction option. Moreover, at the moment one cannot give up one's right to reproduce by cloning, but one can give up the right to use a surrogate mother. The reason is that human

reproductive cloning is so far at the stage of scientific probability, and it is not at all certain that it will ever move to the
stage of possibility. So, for the time being, what one can only
claim – given the current state of affairs with respect to human
reproductive cloning – is the right to hope that cloning will
one day become a reproductive possibility. It is clear, however,
that invoking the right to some hope or probability, while not
unreasonable or *prima facie* objectionable, is not as strong as
invoking the right to a corresponding tangible possibility or
reality. Invoking the right to procreate through cloning could
be compared, *mutatis mutandis*, to invoking the right to free
transportation by astral travel: All indications are that astral
travel will be offered as a possibility in the near or distant future, but it is not the case today. If, for some reason, NASA or
other relevant organizations were to stop research and thus
make the possibility of interstellar travel a distant prospect,
my claim that this would violate my right to free transportation would be quite problematic. In any case, it would not
have the same validity as the corresponding claim if I were
arbitrarily and unjustifiably denied access to air or train travel
today. Rights of any kind are reasonable and valid claims of
the moral person to *something*.[254] However, for the claim to
be reasonable and strong, that *something* must exist and be
offered as a possibility.[255] Otherwise, the relevant discussion
can only be contingent. Considering that human reproductive

---

[254] For an early discussion on claiming a right to something that nevertheless
is not an option, see John S. Mackenzie, "Rights and Duties," *International
Journal of Ethics* 6, no. 4 (1896): 425-441, esp. 432ff. For the limitations
of rights see Phillip Montague, "The Nature of Rights: Some Logical
Considerations," *Noûs* 19, no. 3 (1985): 365-377.

[255] Herbert Lionel Adolphus Hart, *Essays on Bentham: Studies in Jurisprudence
and Political Theory* (Oxford: Clarendon Press, 1982), 185: "Thus, it is hard
to think about rights except as capable of *exercise* [...]"

cloning is still today just probable, I think that invoking the right to reproduce by cloning today is at least premature, if not completely pointless.

Apart from this, according to many contemporary thinkers, those who invoke the right to reproductive freedom as a human rather than a purely moral right, while treating it as absolute and unconditional, confuse the function of the former with that of the latter. Moral rights, by definition, derive from a particular worldview and moral stance, apply primarily at the interpersonal level, and can be either absolute or relative. As noted above, however, human rights are directed not so much at individuals as at states, organizations, etc.[256] Moreover, their enforcement and exercise are inherently subject to conditions and limitations that are rarely present in the case of moral rights.[257] In particular, to say that X has a moral right to P (or to have P happen) is to say that X has a claim on something over another Ψ. Ψ, in turn, if she acknowledges the validity of this claim, describes for herself the corresponding moral obligation to bring her behavior in line with X's right to P. However, the proposition that X possesses the human right to P (or to have P happen) does not presuppose the existence of another Ps, but of many Ps who are largely free to decide to what extent, in what ways, and under what conditions they will respond to X's claim, even though they may in fact recognize it as valid. For example, when I explain to someone that I have a right to know the truth about a matter of mutual concern, I invoke my moral right to know the truth in return for my interlocutor's moral obligation to tell me the truth on the basis of a common agreement between us, or a shared frame of reference, a mutually acceptable

[256] Thomas Pogge, "The International Significance of Human Rights," *Journal of Ethics* 4 (2000): 47.

[257] See George Annas, "Human Cloning," *American Bar Association Journal* 83 (1997): 80-81.

moral code that requires, among other things, that we always
tell each other the truth. If my interlocutor wants to remain
faithful to this shared ethical code of conduct, she must tell me
the truth, regardless of her own inclination, circumstances, best
interests, etc. The same is not true, however, when I invoke, for
example, my human right to health, which is described in the
twenty-fifth article of the First Declaration of Human Rights.
The invocation of this right is intended, on the one hand, to
shape the attitude not of another moral person but of a state
or intergovernmental body. On the other hand, the respect for
this right by the State in which I live is subject to the limitations that the public interest,[258] existing opportunities, as well
as other circumstances, may always impose and that relativize
this right, especially in cases of conflict.[259] My right to health
may have a high value,[260] but this is by no means absolute. On
the contrary, it always depends on other parameters: It is limited by the capacity of the state in which I live (which may not
be able to provide me with health services), by the priorities of
society as a whole (which may dictate that the available health
services should be used not by me but by someone else with a
longer life expectancy), etc.[261] In other words, while it is difficult
to override my right to health care, it is possible to do so for

---

[258] See Robert Nozick, *Anarchy, State and Utopia* (Oxford: Blackwell, 1974),
28-33.

[259] Judith Jarvis Thomson, *The Realm of Rights* (Cambridge, MA: Oxford
University Press, 1990), esp. 158ff.

[260] Maurice Cranston, "Human Rights, Real and Supposed," in *Political
Theory and the Rights of Man*, ed. David Raphael, 43-53 (London: Macmillan,
1967), 52: "A human right is something of which no one should be deprived
without a grave affront to justice."

[261] This view also supports the individual's right to reproductive freedom.
One of the most prominent advocates of this right, Ronald Dworkin, defines
the right to *reproductive autonomy* as "a right to control their own role in
procreation *unless the state has a compelling reason for denying them that*

more serious and important reasons.[262] The human right to reproduction or the right to reproductive freedom, therefore, can only be subject to the same restrictions.[263]

To sum up, the right to reproductive freedom, whether we consider it a purely moral right or a human right, cannot be considered absolute or unlimited for various reasons (for some, this may also mean that the right to reproductive freedom cannot be considered a proper human right at all). On the contrary, when it conflicts with other equally weighty – or even more weighty – moral imperatives, or when broader interests are at stake, it can be either overridden or suspended, but without being invalidated. Thus, invoking the right to reproductive freedom, even with regard to people for whom cloning is the only chance to have biologically related offspring, such as same-sex couples or individuals, does not appear to be as effective as it is thought to be with regard to human reproductive cloning.

III. Being discernible

Human cloning by means of somatic cell nuclear transfer is controversial mainly because it is assumed that it can be used to create a new human being who would be thoroughly identical to another, the prototype, as has already been done with other non-human mammals, most notably Dolly the sheep.

---

control" [emphasis mine]. See Ronald Dworkin, *Life's Dominion* (London: Harper Collins, 1993), 148.

[262] Griffin, 314.

[263] Harris, "Goodbye Dolly? The Ethics of Human Cloning," 359: "In so far as decisions to reproduce […] constitute decisions concerning central issues of value, then arguably the freedom to make them is guaranteed by the constitution (written or not) of any democratic society, unless the state has a compelling reason for denying its citizens that control. To establish such a compelling reason the state […] would have to show that more was at stake […]."

However, this raises an unprecedented and equally serious moral concern: Human cloning will inevitably result in two absolutely identical human beings who will share the same social environment for at least part of their lives and will probably have to live in the closest possible proximity. This is indeed a quite plausible hypothesis, since cloning is likely to be a reproductive option for infertile couples or individuals who desire biologically related offspring. It is certain that in most cases clones and their prototypes[264] will relate to each other in the same way that parents relate to their children or siblings relate to each other. The fact that clones are genetic copies that must live with their prototypes for at least part of their lives will, in the view of many ethicists, inevitably burden clones in ways that non-clones generally are not burdened: In particular, some argue that clones' right to uniqueness or individuality will be compromised, a right that all humans inherently enjoy, and that this will place a heavy psychological burden on the clone.

On March 13, 1997, the European Parliament in its resolution on human cloning decided to ban human cloning research in the European Union and called on the United Nations to take all necessary measures to enact a clear and universal legally binding ban on human cloning. The European Parliament stressed "that each individual has a right to his or her own genetic identity and that human cloning is, and must continue to be, prohibited."[265] This formulation reflects, first, the belief

---

[264] The term *prototype* is used here instead of the more correct terms *genetic prototype* or *donor of genetic material* for reasons of consistency with the hitherto prevailing terminology. Whenever it is used in the following, this will be for the same reasons. However, I do not at all subscribe to the notion that a human clone, if one is ever created, will be a *copy of* another human being in anything other than, perhaps, its phenotype.

[265] The European Parliament, "Resolution on Cloning," *Official Journal C*

that human beings do indeed have an individual genetic identity, second, that this is a human right, and finally, that cloning would violate this right for one category of human beings, the clones, which would diminish their value as human beings as a whole.[266] As Arthur Caplan argues in this context,

> one of the things we treasure about ourselves is our individuality [...]. You begin to worry that when you deliberately set out to make copies of something, you lessen its worth.[267]

In copying and genome editing there is a risk that the clone will lose either its uniqueness,[268] i.e., its individual genetic identity,[269] or the *sense of* being unique. As Dan Brock notes these two risks are related but not identical.[270] I will deal with the second risk, the loss of a sense of uniqueness, in detail in a later chapter. In this chapter, I will focus on the extent to which the right to uniqueness is actually compromised.

It is clear that the argument invoking the clone's right to uniqueness, which is thought to be affected precisely because of the way the clone is created, treats uniqueness as a qualitative and not a quantitative parameter, since the clone and its prototype are two beings and not one.[271] Thus, in the context of the

---

034 02/02/1998, 0164.

[266] Ahlberg, and Brighouse, 541.

[267] Cited by Ruth Macklin in "Splitting Embryos on the Slippery Slope: Ethics and Public Policy," *Kennedy Institute of Ethics Journal* 4, no. 3 (1994): 215.

[268] Kathinka Evers, "The Identity of Clones," *Journal of Medicine and Philosophy* 24, no. 1 (1999): 74.

[269] Macklin, 215.

[270] Dan Brock, "Human Cloning and Our Sense of Self," *Science* 296 (2002): 314.

[271] Ibid.

argument discussed here, human uniqueness is associated with a unique and unrepeatable genome,[272] or the genotype of the individual is associated with both its phenotype and personality, a concept commonly referred to as *genetic determinism*. However, genetic determinism is highly controversial in terms of its consistency, on the one hand, and its scope and applicability, on the other. Nevertheless, the validity of genetic determinism is not the only parameter that is controversial with respect to the argument discussed here. Controversial, moreover, are [a] the extent to which cloning can create two individuals with identical genomes, [b] whether and to what extent the genotype, even if indeed absolutely common to the clone and its prototype, necessarily leads to shared phenotypic expressions, and [c] the hypothesis that an identical genotype necessarily leads to shared personality and character traits – this is what I defined earlier as genetic determinism. However, the objections are not limited to the realm of science. Several ethicists have contributed to the debate with arguments aimed at [d] the possibility that two different beings can be absolutely identical, [e] the possibility of accepting such a right as that to uniqueness, and [f] the view that creating an organism identical to another, even if this were possible, would actually harm the clone or violate the clone's rights.

As for [a] the assumed genetic identity between the clone and the prototype, it is often pointed out that this is by no means self-evident and may even be impossible. This is because in cloning, the nucleus of the somatic cell of the prototype is necessarily introduced into a nucleated oocyte that is different from the oocyte that was fertilized when the prototype was created. However, the oocyte contributes significant-

---

[272] Dan Brock, "Cloning Human Beings: An Assessment of the Ethical Issues Pro and Con," in *Cloning and the Future of the Human Embryo Research*, ed. Paul Lauritzen, 93-113 (New York: Oxford University Press, 2001), 103.

ly to shaping the genetic structure of the created human, as the cytoplasm of the mother cell transfers both cellular and mitochondrial DNA,[273] with an overall contribution to the created genome of 0.05 percent.[274] This difference is not negligible, especially when one considers that minor gene differences lead to significant phenotypic variation, as is the case with homozygous twins. Thus, it is obvious that the clone will differ even slightly from its prototype in DNA structure, to a far greater extent "than the degree to which homozygous twins derived from the same nucleus and cytoplasm differ from each other."[275] Consequently, the clones will differ from their prototypes in terms of genetic specificity and thus will be genetically *unique.*

As for [b] whether common genotypes must necessarily lead to common phenotypes, this view is contested on the basis of existing scientific experience with humans born as nonclones. In particular, it has been observed that genes do not remain stable, but are subject to constant mutations,[276] as random factors and the peculiarities of each prenatal environment make it arbitrary which of the genes present are expressed and which are not – leading us to expect genetic differentiation not only between the clone and its prototype, but also between several clones of one and the same prototype.[277] The environment of the uterus influences the phenotype to a considerable extent, which means that it could be expected that the clone would differ from its prototype only due to the corresponding phenotypic varia-

---

[273] Kuhse, 21.

[274] Françoise Baylis, "Human Cloning: Three Mistakes and an Alternative," *Journal of Medicine and Philosophy* 27, no. 3 (2002): 324-325.

[275] Martin LaBar, "The Pros and Cons of Human Cloning," *Thought* 59 (1984): 325.

[276] Baylis, 324-325.

[277] Rollin, 63.

tions, as the clone would develop either in a different uterus or in the same uterus – but with such a time lag that intrauterine conditions will not be uniform.[278] Also, the stages of placentation and development of the embryonic-maternal circuit will undoubtedly be different in the clone than in its prototype embryo, for they differ even in identical twins developing simultaneously in the same uterus, suggesting even greater differences in clonal appearance than are observed in identical twins.[279] Even greater differences can be expected in the brain structure of the clone compared with that of the prototype, because at the molecular level the neural network is so complex that it is impossible to obtain two identical neural networks, even if the gene set is identical.[280] As Pence notes,

> The conclusion is inescapable: the problem of wiring up a brain is so complex, that it is beyond the power of the genomic computer. The best the genes can do is indicate the rough layout of the wiring, the general shape of the brain. Neurons in this early stage, are thrown together more or less at random and then left to their own devices. After birth, experience makes and brakes connections, pruning the thicket into precise circuity. From the very beginning what's in the genes is different from what's in the brain. And the gulf continues to widen as the brain matures.[281]

---

[278] Baylis, 324-325.

[279] Leon Eisenberg, "The Outcome as Cause: Predestination and Human Cloning," *The Journal of Medicine and Philosophy* 1, no. 4 (1976): 324.

[280] Ngan Tina Huang, "The Ethics of Human Genetic Cloning," *MIT Undergraduate Research Journal* 4 (2001): 70.

[281] Gregory E. Pence, *Who's Afraid of Human Cloning?* (New York: Rowman and Littlefield, 1998), 14.

It should also be noted that the human brain is formed to a considerable extent after the birth of the individual and therefore the

> elaboration of pathways and interconnections is highly dependent on the quantity, quality, and timing of intellectual and emotional stimulation. […] The richer the environment, the greater the complexity of dendritic branching and synaptic junctions and the more efficient the learning when the animal is exposed to novel situations.[282]

As Eisenberg notes, phenotypic identity requires both a shared genome and a shared environment.[283] As it turns out, however, neither the first nor the second condition appears to be satisfied in the case of clones. Thus, contrary to the widespread assumption that the clone and its prototype resemble each other like two drops of water in terms of their genetic makeup and phenotype, this seems quite unlikely. Thus, at the level of genetic and physical similarity, the clone's right to uniqueness does not seem to be violated.

As for [c] personality and character, it is only within the framework of the strictest genetic determinism that one could accept that both are determined in all their aspects and manifestations by one's genetic makeup. On the contrary, the contribution of the environment – familial, social, historical, cultural – in which each of us develops, is perhaps more important than the contribution of our genetic nature to the formation of our

---

[282] Eisenberg, 324-325.

[283] Ibid., 324.

character and personality.[284] This can be seen in the differences
– sometimes striking – in the personality and character of homozygous twins, even though they develop in the closest possible proximity to each other. But even this is not enough to make
their character and personality identical – in fact, homozygous
twins are usually very different in this respect: It seems that
even weak differences in the spatial and temporal position one
occupies are capable of producing significant differences in the
way one perceives one's environment and oneself, one's worldview in general – and, of course, one's personality.[285] Precisely because twins are *two beings* and not *one*, their experiences,
which contribute greatly to the formation of their personalities,
cannot possibly be common,[286] even if they are due to the same
stimuli. As Kathinka Evers notes,

> Every living organism occupies a unique location
> in space and time; each life constitutes a unique
> spatio-temporal sequence. This makes individual
> experience unique and, strictly speaking, impos-
> sible to share. A person can tell another about her
> experiences, but the other can never live them,
> being "bound" elsewhere, imprisoned in another
> spatio-temporal region, and therefore unable to
> view the first person's perspective from within.[287]

In the case of clones, not even the closeness that exists between
homozygous twins is to be expected, for clones will at best

---

[284] Ahlberg, and Brighouse, 541.

[285] Nestor Micheli Morales, "Psychological Aspects of Human Cloning and
Genetic Manipulation: The Identity and Uniqueness of Human Beings,"
Ethics, Bioscience and Life 4, no. 3 (2009): 44.

[286] Rollin, 62.

[287] Evers, 72.

be delayed twins, while they can always arise in a completely different time and place than their prototype – it is to be expected that their experiences will be completely different. This will result in them – the clones – being completely different persons than their prototypes, far more different than identical twins are from each other or children from their parents; by the way, identical twins are already so different that no one can really believe – and no one actually claims that this is the case – that they are not unique. It is also downright absurd to assume that clones – many of whom will be more than twenty years removed from their originals – will experience the same historical events, develop in the same cultural environment, or even experience the same unexpected vicissitudes of fate by which each individual's personality is determined. In light of all this, it seems that the similarity of the genetic makeup of two individuals is far from sufficient to imply identification in terms of character and personality. Leon Eisenberg summarizes this view:

> To produce another Mozart, we would need not only Wolfgang's genome but mother Mozart's uterus, father Mozart's music lessons, their friends and his, the state of music in eighteenth-century Austria, Hayden's patronage, and on and on, in ever-widening circles. Without his set of genes, the rest would not suffice; there has been, after all, only one Wolfgang Amadeus Mozart. But we have no right to the converse assumption: that his genome, cultivated in another world at another time, would result in an equally creative musical genius.[288]

---

[288] Eisenberg, 326.

The conclusion that scientists seem to reach, namely that there is no chance that the clone will be completely identical to the prototype in terms of genotype, phenotype, and personality – or at least *so* similar as to violate the clone's right to uniqueness – is also drawn by philosophers. However, they arrive at this conclusion in different ways. Kathinka Evers, in particular, resorts to an analytical disambiguation of the notion of uniqueness, even invoking Leibniz's famous axiom about the *identity of the indiscernibles*, to prove that [d] the uniqueness of clones is not affected in the case of human cloning. In Evers' view, the assumption that cloning should produce completely identical individuals suffers from the ambiguity that characterizes the concept of identity as used in the context of the argument considered here. Identity, by definition, can be understood as either a quantitative or a qualitative concept. In the first case, we refer to quantities that are numerically identical, such as two weeks of the year that are identical in terms of the number of days they consist of. In this case, we speak of *identical* sets. In the second meaning, identity refers to qualities. In this case we speak of *indiscernible* sets. And given that cloning, by definition, aims at creating at least a second being, the identification of the clone with the prototype can only be understood in this second meaning of the term, i.e., as the absolute identity of the qualities and properties of the clone with those of its prototype. Consequently, the clone and its prototype are identical in the sense that the former cannot be distinguished from the latter.[289] However, the possibility that two beings are indistinguishable in terms of their qualities or properties, that is, that they are indistinguishable but not identical, that is, that they can be distinguished numerically but not qualitatively, has been questioned. In other words, many hold that two beings cannot have all prop-

---

[289] Evers, 69.

erties in common unless they are in fact not two beings but *one*.[290] Or, to put it more simply, there is no way that two different beings can have all their properties in common. Leibniz formulated the above axiom as follows: "[...] it is not true that two substances can resemble each other completely, and differ only in number (*solo numero*)."[291] Elsewhere Leibniz goes into even more detail:

> From these considerations it also follows that, in nature, there cannot be two individual things that differ in number alone. For it certainly must be possible to explain why they are different, and that explanation must derive from some difference they contain. And so what St. Thomas recognized concerning separated intelligences, which, he said, never differ by number alone, must also be said of other things, for never do we find two eggs or two leaves or two blades of grass in a garden that are perfectly similar. And thus, perfect similarity is found only in incomplete and abstract notions, where things are considered only in a certain respect, but not in every way, as, for example, when we consider shapes alone, and neglect the matter that has shape.[292]

---

[290] For an insightful discussion on the issue, see Dieter Birnbacher, "Copying and the Limits of Substitutability," in *The Aesthetics of and Ethics of Copying*, eds. Darren Hudson Hick, and Reinold Schmücker, 3-18 (London: Bloomsbury Academic, 2016), where Birnbacher discusses the case of *Amphitryon* to explore the possibility of creating a perfect identity copy.

[291] Gottfried W. F. von Leibniz, *Discourse on Metaphysics and Other Essays*, trans. Daniel Garber, and Roger Ariew (Indianapolis, and Cambridge: Hackett, 1991), 9.

[292] Gottfried W. F. von Leibniz, "Primary Truths," in *Philosophical Essays*, trans. Roger Ariew, and Daniel Garber (Indianapolis: Hackett, 1989), 32. The reference to St. Thomas Aquinas is from his *Summa Theologica* I, q. 50, art. 4.

In other words, if two beings or objects are to be distinguished from each other numerically, there must be *at least* one qualitative difference between them: If, for any property *F*, *x is* distinguished by *F* if and only if *y* is also distinguished by *F*, then *x* is identical with *y*. This axiom, commonly called Leibniz's *law of the identity of the indiscernibles* can, of course, be reversed following the law of contraposition, leading to McTaggart's *law of the dissimilarity of the diverse*: If *x* and *y are* numerically distinct, then there is at least one property *F* that *x* possesses but *y* does not, and vice versa. McTaggart writes:

> Can there, then, be two things which are exactly similar? I think that the answer must be that there cannot. The connection between diversity and dissimilarity is, no doubt, synthetic. "A and B are two things," and "A and B are dissimilar," are not two ways of stating the same fact. But it seems clear to me that diversity implies dissimilarity – that two things cannot have the same nature. If we make the experiment of removing in thought all difference of nature from two substances, we shall find that, when we have succeeded, we are no longer contemplating two substances, but one.[293]

So, to return to the discussion of cloning, the clone and the prototype can only differ in their characteristics and qualities, and that is the definition of uniqueness. No matter how much faith one places in genetic determinism and its views, therefore, it is always faulty logic to insist that the uniqueness of clones be questioned on the basis of absolute genotypic or phenotypic identity with prototypes.

---

[293] McTaggart, vol. 1, §94.

But even if we accept this, and even though there will be no absolute genotypic and phenotypic identity of the clone with the prototype or similarities in personality with the original, there remains the possibility that the similarity between the clone and the prototype will be such that the clone's right to uniqueness will be violated. However, several ethicists question [e]the possibility of recognizing such a right – at least in the way its proponents seem to understand it – and the reasons given are particularly valid. If there were such a right, it would apply not in all cases, but only to persons who are not born as identical twins. At this point, it should be noted that the rate of identical twin pregnancies is 1:270, which means that in a population of, say, sixty million people, about two hundred thousand people are identical twins.[294] However, we are far from assuming that all these people, because they are born as identical twins, are deprived of any right that other people enjoy. If that were the case, we should at least pity identical twins for the injustice – or misfortune – they have to suffer. But neither do we treat them that way, nor do twins seem to perceive themselves as non-unique beings or as moral persons who have fewer rights because they are twins.

Nature spontaneously produces her own clones, and since no one believes that they are deprived of their right to uniqueness, there is no reason to believe otherwise in the case of *artificial twins*. According to Harris,

> artificial clones raise no difficulty which is not already raised by the phenomenon of natural twins. We are not alarmed when natural twins are born – why should we be alarmed when they are deliberately created?[295]

---

[294] Harris, "Goodbye Dolly? The Ethics of Human Cloning," 356.
[295] Ibid., 353.

Of course, one could object by claiming that natural processes cannot interfere with moral rights, only human actions can do this: When someone is struck by lightning and killed, we do not normally think that her right to life has been violated, unless we think metaphysically. However, if a human being is killed by another human being, under certain circumstances we may think that her right to life has been violated. Similarly, when nature creates clones. Even if, by virtue of being born as clones, they are ultimately deprived of the uniqueness by which all other human beings are distinguished, it makes no sense to assume that the clone's right to uniqueness has been violated in case of naturally born identical twins; but we are entitled to think that this is the case when clones are intentionally created. This reasoning, while plausible, is nevertheless unconvincing. After all, the birth of natural twins can be sought and achieved by human action without this in turn being considered a violation of the natural twins' right to uniqueness. Especially in the context of various assisted reproduction techniques – and assisted reproduction, mind you, is often considered a human right[296] – multiple pregnancy is very likely, as more than two fertilized eggs are implanted in the mother's uterus to ensure success. Very often – more often than in nature – assisted reproduction results in multiple pregnancies. Although assisted reproduction could be considered in this sense as the intentional creation of twins or triplets, no one considers that the right to uniqueness is violated in the case of these children.[297] The result is that either the right to uniqueness makes no sense at all or that it cannot be violated because of genotypic and phenotypic similarity. Dan Brock goes even further and takes the position that invoking

---

[296] See the previous chapter on the *Right to Reproductive Freedom*.

[297] Brock, "Cloning Human Beings: An Assessment."

this right in the context of cloning is merely an anachronism that is difficult to justify, since

> The idea of the uniqueness, or unique identity, of each person historically predates the development of modern genetics and the knowledge that except in the case of homozygous twins, each individual has a unique genome. A unique genome thus could not be the grounds of this long-standing belief in the unique human identity of each person.[298]

It is clear from the discussion so far that invoking the danger that the clone's right to uniqueness will be violated because the clone is a copy[299] of an existing or pre-existing human being is not a valid argument. This is because all the concepts that form the premises of the argument are highly controversial, sometimes in terms of their content and sometimes in terms of their relevance to the question under consideration. In addition, it is also controversial [f] whether the creation of a clone, even if it were possible, would actually harm the clone or violate its rights, since the child that would be born as a clone could not have been created in any way other than as clone. This is commonly referred to as the *non-identity problem*, which I will discuss later.[300]

IV. Not knowing one's own genetic makeup

It is often argued that the clone, as a genetic copy or later twin of an already existing human being, would have more – possibly complete – knowledge about her genetic characteristics

---

[298] Ibid., 104.

[299] The same applies to the use of the term *copy as to* the term *original*. See note 128.

[300] See the chapter on the *Right to an open future*.

than other humans. Since everyone's future is to some extent genetically predetermined, the clone has much more data about herself and her future than any other human whose birth did not occur through reproductive cloning. For example, when the clone looks at her 'prototype,' she will know approximately what she will look like when she reaches the age of the human from whom her genetic material was taken. She will also know what diseases or conditions are likely to affect her, what predispositions she has, and in some cases, she will even be able to determine her life expectancy. She will not be able to discover herself as any other person could because she already knows too much about herself. If we assume that the ability to discover oneself during life is an ongoing event that gives value to life, then the clone seems to suffer an undue and unwarranted harm by being born as such. At the same time, partial knowledge of her future, however uncertain or inaccurate, distinguishes her from other humans in a way that may be psychologically stressful to the clone. When this is the case, it appears that the clone suffers a special and undeserved harm by the nature of her creation. Knowledge of her genetic peculiarities, her genetic structure, and what that structure predicts for her future can also be a stressful and damaging psychological event. For example, imagine that your genetic structure describes a trivial but real possibility of a degenerative brain disease such as Alzheimer's or some form of cancer. You will most likely spend your entire life fearing the phenotypic realization of your genetic predisposition, but it may remain at the level of probability until the end of your life. This knowledge may cause you to hesitate (probably wrongly) or even refuse when it comes to, for example, committing to a steady partner, starting a family and having offspring, or pursuing a career in a field in which you have the potential to excel, etc. In all these cases and others, you are harmed by the fact that you have come into life as a clone of a person who has preceded you.

Cloning seems to imply for the clone a knowledge of herself so special and profound that it does not seem to be available to any other human being, since no category of human beings other than clones possesses such knowledge. This knowledge, it is often argued, is so staggering that it condemns the clone to spend her life *in the shadow* of her prototype.[301] This is already a direct harm done to the clone and an injustice, since the clone alone bears the burden of this knowledge and, moreover, because of the nature of its creation, cannot escape this burden. To illustrate this unique position of the clone, let me give the following example. Genetic counseling[302] is available today to anyone who wants it and can afford it: One can have one's genome mapped, one's potentially undesirable genetic predispositions revealed, and thus receive advice on what foods to avoid, what activities to engage in, etc., to minimize the risk of those predispositions coming to fruition. Nevertheless, genetic counseling is by no means considered a moral duty for moral agents, but rather a right, and it is left to one's own will whether to seek genetic counseling. Now imagine that my genetic material somehow comes into the possession of laboratory personnel without my knowledge and without my consent; the laboratory personnel examine my genetic material and determine that I am predisposed to a potentially fatal disease, so the director decides to inform me. It would still be my decision whether to accept or reject the information, and the lab director would have to respect my decision, whatever it may be. This duty stems from my right not to know, i.e., the right to refuse medical

---

[301] See Sören Holm, "A Life in the Shadow: One Reason Why We Should Not Clone Humans," *Cambridge Quarterly of Healthcare Ethics* 7 (1998): 160-162.

[302] See Barbara B. Biesecker, "Goals of Genetic Counseling," *Clinical Genetics* 60 (2001): 323-330. For a case related to unintended knowledge,

information about the condition and prospects of my own health, provided, of course, that this does not harm the interests of other people or society as a whole.[303] It seems that in the case of clones the right not to know will be very limited, if it exists at all.

The duty not to disclose information about one's heredity, dispositions, etc., against one's will is based on the value we generally place on self-determination[304] or the autonomy of moral agents – for Kantian ethicists, it is this capacity that enables humans to escape the heteronomy of the phenomenal world and to have free will.[305] However, if moral duties are linked to corresponding moral rights as giving raise to them, then it follows that the duty to respect one's will, to know nothing about one's state of health and future prospects, outlines a corresponding right to ignorance, in this case ignorance of one's genetic constitution. This right to ignorance is compromised when someone gives us information about our genetic makeup against our will. In the case of cloning, many argue that this right is violated from the moment the clone is born, since some information – that can remain unknown to non-clones if they wish to avoid it – is inescapable to clones.

For those who accept such a right – and not all do – the right to genetic ignorance is a negative right. In other words, it describes for those who are in the vicinity of the bearer of this right the duty not to act in such a way as to reveal to her information about her genetic makeup if she does not wish to have such

---

see J. Hogan, A. Turner, K. Tucker, and L. Warwick, "Unintended Diagnosis of Von Hippel Lindau Syndrome Using Array Comparative Genomic Hybridization (CGH): Counseling Challenges Arising from Unexpected Information," *Journal of Genetic Counseling* 22 (2013): 22-26.

[303] Tuija Takala, "The Right to Genetic Ignorance Confirmed," *Bioethics* 13, nos. 3-4 (1999): 289.

[304] Wood, 175.

[305] Juha Raikka, "Freedom and the Right (not) to Know," *Bioethics* 12, no. 1

information. This is because complete ignorance of our genetic nature is impossible, since we all acquire some knowledge of it during our lives, whether we want it or not. But when the relevant information is forced upon us by others against our will, we seem to be offended differently than when we learn, for example, that a distant ancestor of ours suffered from Huntington's disease or that our grandfather had Parkinson's. In these cases, too, we receive information about our genetic predisposition, and this is because these diseases are genetic and therefore hereditary, but because such information comes as a random event, it does not affect the right to ignorance. As Tuija Takala notes,

> Given the fact that people cannot be adequately protected against genetic information in any case – they only need to look in the mirror or meet their blood relatives to know something about their genetic make-up – it would seem that the right to genetic ignorance can only be a negative claim right. By a negative claim right I mean that the right-holder has no duty to know about her own genetic make-up, and that others have a duty not to inform her (against her own wishes).[306]

The inevitable violation of this right in the case of cloning burdens the clone with unwanted knowledge that even identical twins do not possess about themselves.[307] Identical twins, as Hans Jonas notes, have the same genetic material but are born

(1998): 50-51.

[306] Tuija Takala, "The Many Wrongs of Human Reproductive Cloning," in *Bioethics and Social Reality*, eds. Matti Hayry, Tuija Takala, and Peter Herissone-Kelly, 53-66 (Amsterdam, and New York: Rodopi, 2005), 62.

[307] Brock, "Human Cloning and Our Sense of Self," 315.

at the same time and therefore, like all humans, cannot have any foresight into the course of their future lives. Therefore, they are free to shape their lives by choosing spontaneously, freely, and authentically among the possibilities that open up to them each time.[308] For the clone, on the other hand, to the extent that her future is determined by the genomic data with which she is endowed, it would be sufficient to take a look at her 'prototype' or to consult her prototype's medical records in order to gain some measure of knowledge about herself, whether she likes it or not. Such knowledge would undoubtedly make it inevitable that the clone would be forced to live in the shadow of the prototype, at least to some degree.

This feeling of living a life in the shadow of her prototype would undoubtedly be reinforced for the clone by other people's attitudes toward her. According to Sören Holm, a form of genetic determinism (he speaks of *genetic essentialism*) is widespread today,[309] under which it is generally assumed that our genes determine our psychological profile and personality as a whole, and that our selves can be reduced to their molecular structure, so that human beings "in all their social, moral, and historical complexity with the genes that make up their genetic material."[310] This view is reinforced every time scientists announce that they have discovered a gene responsible for depression or schizophrenia, for example.[311] With this in mind, the starting point for clones would be completely different from that of non-clones, and a very disadvantageous one, because the existence of their prototype,

---

[308] Hans Jonas, *Philosophical Essays: From Ancient Creed to Technological Man* (Englewood Cliffs: Prentice-Hall, 1974), 159.

[309] See Holm, 161.

[310] Dorothy Nelkin, and Suzan Lindee, *The DNA Mystique: The Gene as a Cultural Icon* (New York: W.H. Freeman and Company, 1995), 2.

[311] Holm, 161.

> [...] will dictate from the outset to those who
> know – to the clone itself and its environment
> alike – all the expectations, predictions, hopes
> and fears, goals and comparisons, as well as the
> measure of that person's success or failure.[312]

As Holm notes, it is very likely that the 'parents' of the clone, because of their knowledge of the life history of the individual from which the genetic material of the clone was taken, already have a very precise idea of how the clone will develop, which largely determines their behavior toward the clone:

> They will try to prevent some developments,
> and try to promote others. Just imagine how a
> clone of Adolf Hitler or Pol Pot would be reared,
> or how a clone of Albert Einstein, Ludwig van
> Beethoven, or Michael Jordan would be brought
> up. The clone would in a very literal way live his
> or her life in the shadow of the life of the origi-
> nal. At every point in the clone's life there would
> be someone who had already lived that life, with
> whom the clone could be compared and against
> whom the clone's accomplishments could be
> measured.[313]

In this way, Holm argues, the clone's ability to live her own life to the fullest would be limited, as she would be pressured –

---

[312] Hans Jonas, "Lasst uns einen Menschen klonieren: Von der Eugenik zu der Gentechnologie," in his *Technik, Medizin und Ethik – Praxis des Prinzips der Verantwortung* (Frankfurt am Main: Suhrkamp, 1987), 190 [translation from German mine].

[313] Holm, 161.

either by herself or by her environment – to shape her life, in part by following the life of her prototype and trying to avoid its mistakes or achieve its achievements.[314] In either case, then, the clone would have borne an undue burden that no other human being would have had to bear. The burden of having (or being *under the impression* of having) another human being as a point of reference, whose life we are expected to live for some reason and to some degree, is on full display in the dramatic stories of many descendants of Nazi war criminals, some of whom went so far as to voluntarily have themselves sterilized in order to "cut the line" and not allow the "blood of a monster," that of their criminal ancestor, to be passed on to future generations, as Bettina Goering, granddaughter of Hitler's deputy Hermann Goering, explained when she had herself sterilized.[315] It is obvious that she made this decision under the weight of her grandfather's shadow, even though she shared only a small part of her genetic material with him. It is therefore easy to speculate about how much more pronounced the shadow of an individual might be on a clone, if the clone shares not only a small part of this individual's genetic material, but almost all of it.

If the moral value we attach to the autonomy of the moral person and her corresponding capacity for self-determination is due to that these principles enable individuals to possess and exercise the right to live as they wish, then the fact that clones would be partially deprived of this opportunity and forced to live in the shadow of their prototype – apart from being a violation of their right to autonomy and self-determination – would undermine the validity of the fundamental

---

[314] Ibid., 162.

[315] Allan Hall, "Hermann Goering's Great-Niece: I Had Myself Sterilized So I Would Not Pass on the Blood of a Monster," *The Daily Mail*, January 21, 2010.

moral principles on which these rights are based.[316] In other words, the clones' negative moral right to ignorance – which includes the corresponding duty of other moral persons not to feed them unwanted and potentially harmful information about their genetic makeup – would be violated by default by the fact that they were created as clones of another human being. Consequently, clones would not enjoy full moral status because they would be deprived at birth of a basic moral right to which other moral persons are entitled.

It should be noted that the arguments of both Jonas and Holm, which emphasize the risk that clones will end up living their lives in the shadow of their prototypes and, on the basis of that risk, each argue for the so-called right to genetic ignorance, do not depend for their validity on whether the perceptions of the clone or those around her – about the extent to which the genetic constitution predisposes or determines the individual's personality or future – are right or wrong. The fact that the clone is likely or reasonably likely to believe that she knows more about herself and her future than other people, and that she believes that her future is determined by her genome, is sufficient to establish a violation of the clone's right to genetic ignorance. The fact that beliefs resembling genetic determinism are likely to prevail in the clone's environment, regardless of the extent to which those beliefs are right or wrong, also constitutes harm to the clone because she is again forced to live in the shadow of her prototype. As Holm notes, the living-in-the-shadow argument is based on a tangible and pervasive reality, namely, that there is a strong tendency in society to adopt the positions of genetic determinism, but not on the scientific correctness or soundness of genetic determinism itself, and to that extent the living-in-the-shadow argument

---

[316] Holm, 162.

is sound. In the case genetic determinism is disproved and rejected within the society, the argument is no longer valid. Holm argues, however, that this will most likely not be the case.[317]

In summary, we can say that the argument about living in the shadow emphasizes the probable fact that the clone's environment will burden her by constantly comparing her with her original, while the argument about the right to ignorance focuses mainly on the existential experiences of the clones themselves as people who have been informed in advance (or believe they have) about their own fate.[318] Those who accept the above two interrelated and complementary arguments and assume that the clone can only live a life in the shadow of her prototype and is born with an already violated right to ignorance, more or less follow the following reasoning: [a] Humans have no moral duty to know their genetic nature. [b] The autonomy of the moral person and her right to self-determination allow (or require) the recognition of a derivative right, namely the right to genetic ignorance. [c]This right is not positive, but negative, i.e., it does not impose on a person's environment the obligation to protect her from relevant knowledge in all cases, but describes the obligation not to inform her against her will. [d] The right to genetic ignorance is not absolute, but relative, i.e., it applies unless there are compelling reasons to suspend or abrogate it (public interest, conflict with the rights of other moral persons, etc.). [e] Its violation constitutes harm to the holder, unless there are sufficiently compelling reasons. [f] Cloning unavoidably abrogates the clone's right to genetic ignorance, since it presupposes that the clone knows its genetic constitution, or part of it, and allows its environment to know it as well. [g] The validity of the argu-

---

[317] Ibid., 162.

[318] Takala, "The Many Wrongs," 61.

ment is not affected by the extent to which genetic determinism is true, i.e., whether accurate inferences about the clone's life course or personality can actually be drawn from the clone's genetic makeup, either by the clone herself or by her environment. For this right to be violated, it is sufficient if either the clone or her environment believe that they can draw accurate conclusions about her life course or personality from her genotype, in other words, if they accept the theses of genetic determinism.[319]

Therefore, human reproductive cloning [1] harms the clone by depriving her of a right that all other human beings have and condemns her to a life in the shadow of her prototype, [2] calls into question the value of the principles on which the right to genetic ignorance is based, namely, the autonomy of persons and their capacity for self-determination, [3] creates an inferior class of moral beings, the clones, who, through no fault of their own, possess fewer moral rights than human beings created by ordinary sexual reproduction.[320] It follows from all of this that human reproductive cloning can be considered at best morally problematic.

However, invoking the right to ignorance and projecting the risk that the clone will be forced to live her life in the shadow of her prototype are not irrefutable arguments for considering human reproductive cloning morally problematic. In particular, the validity of the right to ignorance has been questioned both in its theoretical core and in the way it is used in the ethical debate over cloning. In other words, several ethicists argue that such a right either cannot be justified at all, or that, if it can be, it offers no argument in the case of human reproductive cloning.

As to the core of the argument, it has been argued that autonomy, which is predominantly invoked as the theoretical basis

---

[319] Brock, "Human Cloning and Our Sense of Self," 315.

[320] Helga Kuhse, 20.

of the right to genetic ignorance, is violated rather than protected by ignorance, whereas knowledge, on the contrary, guarantees the autonomy of the moral person. Ignorance is by definition a natural state of the human being, conditioned by the finitude of her nature. Equally natural is man's opposite tendency to strive for knowledge: Aristotle begins his *Metaphysics* with the iconic phrase *Πάντες ἄνθρωποι τοῦ εἰδέναι ὀρέγονται φύσει*, that is, "All men naturally desire knowledge."[321] The indisputable fact that the desire for knowledge is a natural human tendency, as well as the equally indisputable fact that knowledge is generally considered useful, beneficial, and good, while ignorance is the opposite, are not sufficient grounds for denying someone her right to ignorance, for she could argue that, on the basis of her free will and autonomy, which make her a moral agent, she prefers to be ignorant rather than knowledgeable in some cases – in this case, about her own genetic makeup. So, the question arises: Can the right to ignorance be sufficiently grounded in the autonomy of moral agents? I will attempt to provide a satisfactory answer to this question by examining it in light of the views of two philosophers whose positions are often invoked by those concerned with bioethics, namely Immanuel Kant and John Stuart Mill.

Kant's general attitude toward ignorance – especially voluntary ignorance – can be effortlessly deduced from his short essay entitled *What is Enlightenment?* Already in the preface to his essay, Kant praises Enlightenment because, by placing knowledge at the top of the hierarchy of values – the spirit of the Enlightenment can be crystallized, according to Kant, in the phrase *sapere aude*, that is, "dare to know" – it freed the human being from the tutelage of ignorance that she had imposed upon herself. For Kant, deliberately impeding the progress of knowledge is an unthinkable decision:

---

[321] Aristotle, *Metaphysics*, 980a 21.

> One age cannot [...] put the next in such a state
> that it cannot advance knowledge, restore it from
> error [...] This would be a crime against human
> nature, whose proper destiny lies precisely in this
> progress. Therefore, succeeding ages are fully
> entitled to repudiate such decisions as unautho-
> rized and outrageous.[322]

If the proper destiny of human nature is the constant development of knowledge, for human beings themselves their destiny
is nothing other than their autonomy, which, according to Kant,
is "the ground of the dignity of human and every other rational
nature,"[323] and "the sole principle of morals."[324] In Kant's thought,
autonomy consists in the freedom of the will and is twofold: In its
negative sense, it is freedom *from* something – the laws of nature,
the will of another, our passions and inclinations, heteronomy in
general – while in its positive dimension it is freedom *to* something, that is, "this quality, to determine itself to action under the
idea of its freedom."[325] As Kant so aptly puts it: "What else, then,
could the freedom of the will be, except autonomy, i.e., the quality
of the will of being a law to itself?"[326]

Nevertheless, every rational nature cannot but succumb to
the view "That all maxims ought to harmonize from one's own
legislation into a possible realm of ends as a realm of nature,"[327]

[322] Immanuel Kant, "What is Enlightenment?" in Immanuel Kant, *Perpetual Peace and Other Essays*, trans. Ted Humphrey, 41-48 (Indianapolis: Hackett Publishing Company, 1983), 8:39.

[323] Kant, *Groundwork for the Metaphysics of Morals*, 4:436.

[324] Ibid., 4:440.

[325] Ibid., 4:448.

[326] Ibid., 4:447.

[327] Ibid., 4:436.

i.e., that they should "judge their actions always in accordance with those maxims of which they themselves can will that they should serve as universal laws."[328] In other words: Whenever the moral agent is asked to choose between two or more possible maxims, she should ask herself: "Which of the maxims among which I can now choose could I wish to become a universal law?" It is obvious that one cannot wish for a maxim that promotes voluntary ignorance to be elevated to universal law – that is, if the possibility of knowledge exists, but I will explain this below. As for the autonomy of the moral agent, it is clear that if the moral person is to decide freely about her moral choices, she must make *informed* and *reality-based* choices. Otherwise, her will is subject to another, subtle and tricky kind of heteronomy: Ignorance is also a condition by which the autonomy of the moral agent is constrained. One might note, of course, that the moral agent can never have all the information necessary to make a decision, and this is because human nature imposes its own limitations – the will of humans remains thus subject to heteronomy due to ignorance in any case. However, it is one thing not to know what has not yet revealed itself to one because of the limitations of one's nature, and another thing to choose to remain ignorant, even though one has the capacity to know. As Rosamond Rhodes notes about the pursuit of (genetic) ignorance,

> As sovereign over myself I am obligated to make thoughtful and informed decisions without being swayed by irrational emotions, including my fear of knowing significant genetic facts about myself. When I recognize that I am ethically required to be autonomous, I must also see that, since autonomous action requires being informed of what

---

[328] Ibid., 4:426.

a reasonable person would want to know under the circumstance, I am ethically required to be informed. So, if I have an obligation to learn what I can, when genetic information is likely to make a significant difference in my decisions and when the relevant information is obtainable with reasonable effort, I have no right to remain ignorant. From the recognition of my own autonomy, I have a duty to be informed. I have no right to remain ignorant.[329]

Our refusal to examine some of the data available to us for choosing our actions simply shows that our will is not free in the negative sense of the term: It is subject to extraneous determination by an irrational passion, the unjustified unwillingness to know important genetic data about ourselves. To the extent that our will is not free, we cannot be autonomous, at least not in the sense in which Kant understands autonomy. If,

The principle of autonomy is thus: 'Not to choose otherwise than so that the maxims of one's choice are at the same time comprehended with it in the same volition as universal law,'[330]

it follows that I must at least have a reasonable belief that the maxim I choose at a given moment could take effect as a universal law, so that my choice is autonomous. Would it be legitimate, however, to claim that someone who deliberately ignores some or all the information that would influence her

---

[329] Rosamond Rhodes, "Genetic Links, Family Ties, and Social Bonds: Rights and Responsibilities in the Face of Genetic Knowledge," *Journal of Medicine and Philosophy* 23, no. 1 (1998): 18.

[330] Kant, *Groundwork for the Metaphysics of Morals*, 4:440.

choice, could reasonably believe that her choice could become a universal law? Such an assertion would be as untenable as someone insisting that she is reasonably convinced that the book she holds in her hands is excellent, even though she has not yet read a single page and knows nothing else about the author or the contents of the book.

Mill, on the other hand, does not speak of autonomy, but of *freedom* and *individuality*.[331] The way he seems to understand these two concepts, however, brings him close – probably, too close – to Kant's conception of autonomy in its negative sense, that is, *freedom from something*, which in Mill's case is primarily freedom from state authority and coercion. Specifically, Mill argues that:

> [...] the only purpose for which power can be rightfully exercised over any member of a civilized community, against his will, is to prevent harm to others. His own good, either physical or moral, is not a sufficient warrant. He cannot rightfully be compelled to do or forbear because it will be better for him to do so, because it will make him happier, because, in the opinion of others, to do so would be wise, or even right. [...] Over himself, over his own body and mind, the individual is sovereign.[332]

If, for Mill, freedom means that one may do as one pleases[333] as long as one does not harm others or interfere with their free-

---

[331] For an excellent essay on Mill's view on both, see among others Robert F. Ladenson, "Mill's Conception of Individuality," *Social Theory and Practice* 4, no. 2 (1977): 167-182.

[332] Mill, *On Liberty*, 13.

[333] Ibid., 93.

dom, and if one does not want to know anything about one's own health and future prospects, then is not the disclosure of an unwanted piece of information – provided that nondisclosure harms no one except possibly the person who chooses not to know – an infringement of one's freedom? In my opinion, Mill would not readily accept this view: For him, freedom seems to be inseparable from knowledge. Since it is plausible to assume that one cannot desire something that will certainly prove harmful to oneself, one should at least be informed of the dangers one will run to be able to decide for oneself whether or not to proceed. If circumstances do not permit one to be informed, and if the risk is certain, one is even justified in using force to prevent someone from proceeding without it being a violation of her liberty. In one of the most famous passages in *On Liberty*, Mill writes:

> If either a public officer or any one else saw a person attempting to cross a bridge which had been ascertained to be unsafe, and there were no time to warn him of his danger, they might seize him and turn him back, without any real infringement of his liberty; for liberty consists in doing what one desires, and he does not desire to fall into the river. Nevertheless, when there is not a certainty, but only a danger of mischief, no one but the person himself can judge of the sufficiency of the motive which may prompt him to incur the risk: in this case, therefore (unless he is a child, or delirious, or in some state of excitement or absorption incompatible with the full use of the reflecting faculty), he ought, I conceive, to be only warned of the danger; not forcibly prevented from exposing himself to it.[334]

---

[334] Ibid., 93.

The above passage has become famous because Mill, otherwise an ardent opponent of paternalism, seems to suggest, oddly enough, a form of mild or soft paternalism[335] designed to ensure that individuals are given the ability to "judge of the sufficiency of the motive" and that if they lack this ability for some reason, others will provide it. In this case, our intervention would not only be justified but even required – the individual, Mill argues, "ought to be warned" – and that is because, unlike the person directly involved, we happen to "possess the kind of information on which a reasonable assessment of the act depends."[336] It is obvious that in Mill's thought freedom also depends on the ability to judge whether or not one desires something, and that the ability to judge is also largely determined by the relevant knowledge one possesses, for one cannot desire anything other than what one knows.

As for the theoretical core of an alleged right to ignorance, several ethicists argue that the concepts of ignorance on the one hand, and moral rights on the other are so incompatible that the concept of a right to ignorance is a contradiction in terms. Moral rights are granted primarily – or exclusively – to moral persons. What makes an individual a moral person is her autonomy, that is, the ability to set and evaluate one's own

[335] Also, *soft* or *elastic* paternalism: "in the absence of competing moral factors (such as the paternalized agent's obligations to others) interference is proper only with those: (1) whom we know to lack sufficient ability to make informed and voluntary decisions vis-à-vis the harmful action or omission, or (2) for whom we do not have sufficient evidence of their ability to do such." See William Glod, "How not to Argue Against Paternalism," *Reason Papers* 30 (2008): 7; also Raphael Cohen-Almagor, "Between Autonomy and State Regulation: J. S. Mill's Elastic Paternalism," *Philosophy* 87, no. 4 (2012): 559ff.

[336] David E. Ost, "The 'Right' Not to Know," *The Journal of Medicine and Philosophy* 9 (1984): 306.

ends and to choose the means to achieve those ends. Autonomy can be limited either by external or internal factors: In the first case, by the imposition of others or by the limitations of the human nature; in the second case, by our inability to function as rational beings.[337] The question of whether ignorance can promote autonomy and agency has already been discussed. We must now consider the extent to which appealing to ignorance is consistent with reason. For, as David Ost notes,

> [...] if we prove that our refusal to receive information is unreasonable, we will have proved that there is no such right. For if this kind of refusal is irrational, and if irrationality is a condition that removes autonomy, and if autonomy constitutes the theoretical basis of rights, then our refusal to receive information *ipso facto* constitutes an acknowledgement that we are not autonomous, i.e., that we cannot be considered as bearers of rights.[338]

But let us now return to Mill's example of the unsuspecting person preparing to cross the unsafe bridge. Suppose that when we finally stopped the person in the example to warn her of the danger she was about to enter, she declared, invoking her right to ignorance, that she did not want to know whether the bridge she was about to cross was safe or not. Her words would indicate that: (a) either no information could have influenced her decision to cross the bridge, or (b) she already has as much information as she needs to make

---

[337] John Harris, and Kirsty Keywood, "Ignorance, Information and Autonomy," *Theoretical Medicine and Bioethics* 22 (2001): 418-419.
[338] Ost, 304.

that decision, including the information you want to give her, but she refuses to accept.

However, as Ost notes, each of these implicit statements would be absurd.[339] The first statement would be the definition of obsession or compulsion, for if no information can influence one's decision, it follows that no information shaped it in the first place and the decision is not rational. The second statement would be self-defeating, because it implies that one can know everything that is relevant to a matter even if one refuses to be informed about everything that is relevant to that matter: The person about to cross the bridge could never be in a position to know all the information she needs to decide whether or not to ultimately cross the bridge, because she does not know the information you would give her if she had not refused your offer. Therefore, her refusal to know the information is indicative of an at least momentarily lapse of reason, which may well be a significant internal constraint on her autonomy. But if the individual is not autonomous, she cannot be considered a moral agent, and she cannot be accorded moral rights, including her right to ignorance. Therefore, according to Ost,

> [...] the contradiction lies in the very recognition of the right [in ignorance] [...] the invocation of the concept of right in this case [...] is inappropriate. To accept the right to ignorance is to accept that the right in question can be recognized in someone who is not a rights-bearer.[340]

---

[339] Ibid., 306.

[340] Ibid., 305.

If ignorance limits autonomy by depriving the moral agent of the opportunity to make informed decisions,[341] and if the pursuit of ignorance raises the question of the extent to which one who pursues ignorance can actually be considered a moral agent and a bearer of rights, then knowledge – in this case about our genetic makeup – seems to enhance and promote human autonomy, especially in the case of genetics, where knowledge, even rudimentary, of any data is extremely unlikely. In many cases, one must make decisions related to one's genetic predisposition, even decisions that can only be made if one has the necessary information about it. For example, if a prospective parent knows that she is a carrier of a serious hereditary disease, she might decide to adopt to avoid the risk that her biological offspring will suffer from the disease of which she is a carrier. She would have good reason to do so, either because of the burden her biological offspring would have to bear if they were born with Huntington's disease, for example, or because of the burden she herself would have to bear as a parent in that case, a burden she may not be willing or able to bear. However, ignorance of her genetic predisposition prevents the carrier of such a genetic disease from deciding for herself whether to take on the risk and the resulting responsibility, thereby limiting her reproductive autonomy, because autonomy generally depends on the possibility of choice, and the possibility of choice in this case presupposes knowledge of her genetic predisposition.[342] Conversely, the ability to make choices based on the relevant genetic data increases the possibility of choice and thus autonomy.

---

[341] Maria Canellopoulou-Bottis, "Comment on a View Favouring Ignorance of Genetic Information: Confidentiality, Autonomy, Beneficence and the Right Not to Know," *European Journal of Health Law* 2 (2000): 185-191.

[342] Graeme Laurie, "Protecting and Promoting Privacy in an Uncertain World: Further Defences of Ignorance and the Right Not to Know," *European Journal of Health Law* 7 (2000): 189.

Advocates of the right not to know one's genetic constitution or condition focus primarily on respect for one's autonomy, in the event that the person wishes to remain in ignorance. Roberto Andorno, in particular, has advocated the right not to know as an exception to both the duty of physicians to inform their patients and the right of patients to know. This exception is justified by the need to preserve confidentiality and privacy and to protect psychologically vulnerable individuals who could suffer great harm if unwanted information is disclosed and who believe it is in their best interest to remain ignorant. As Andorno puts it:

> Precisely one of the particularities of this right consists in the fact that it almost entirely depends on the subjective perceptions of the individual, who is, in fact, the best interpreter of his or her best interest. […] is based on individuals' autonomy and on their interest in not being psychologically harmed by the results of genetic tests.[343]

It is true that today, for various reasons, it is very easy to get one's genetic information. But it is just as easy to pass it on, which on the one hand can lead to knowledge that was not available to people a few generations ago, but on the other hand is also undesirable. Imagine that in a few years genetic tests could show how many years you have left to live. You might not want such knowledge, no matter how irresponsible it might be, and I do not think anyone would blame you. Against this background, I have to admit that introducing a right not to know may seem plausible. On the other hand, establishing it as a typical moral right remains

---

[343] Roberto Andorno, "The Right not to Know: An Autonomy Based Approach," *Journal of Medical Ethics* 30 (2004): 438-439.

problematic. What makes it problematic, in my opinion, is that *ignorance can hardly be understood as a right.* Andorno himself is very careful when it comes to the right not to be informed of the results of genetic testing: It is clear that he does not see this right as unconditional, but that several conditions must be met for it to be binding – the person should be competent, she should have received appropriate genetic counseling,[344] while unlike what is the case with most typical rights, "the right not to know cannot be *presumed*, but should be 'activated' by the explicit will of the person,"[345] and in any case the right not to know remains

> a relative right, in the sense that it may be re-
> stricted when disclosure to the individual is nec-
> essary in order to avoid serious harm to third
> parties, especially family members, which means
> that some form of prevention or treatment is
> available.[346]

In a later essay, Andorno even goes so far as to question the validity of a right not to know in the case of communicable diseases such as HIV, which on the one hand pose a threat to the patient's environment and on the other can be prevented or cured.[347] The upshot is that,

> While autonomous decision making gives us the
> right to refuse to receive burdensome and useless
> information about our genetic makeup, it cannot
> be invoked to remain ignorant of HIV test results

---

[344] Ibid., 438.

[345] Ibid.

[346] Ibid., 439.

[347] Roberto Andorno, "The Right not to Know Does not Apply to HIV Testing," *Journal of Medical Ethics* 42, no. 2 (2016): 104.

when such ignorance would lead us to put the
lives of others at risk.[348]

Tom Beauchamp and James Childress, who also advocate the
right not to know in general, seem to accept the need for information even against one's own will,[349] specifically in the case
where one has a misconception about her condition. Of course,
Beauchamp and Childress are not referring specifically to cloning, but to medical practice in general. However, based on the
above, particularly with respect to genetically transmitted diseases, I believe that their view is valid in this case as well. The
patient who mistakenly believes that the pain from which she
now suffers cannot be controlled in any way, and who therefore, and only therefore, asks for euthanasia, is in no different
position from the prospective parent who mistakenly believes
that she is free from genetically transmissible diseases, and
who therefore chooses to produce natural offspring rather than
adopt, even though she would choose adoption if she knew her
true genetic predisposition. In both cases, knowledge reinforces
the autonomy of the individual by providing her with at least
one additional option and the opportunity to choose it freely
without being constrained by ignorance of the existence of that
option. Thus, if clones do indeed – by virtue of their existence as
such – have more information about their genetic selves, then
their autonomy seems to be enhanced rather than impaired or
constrained. Moreover, as Helga Kuhse notes,

> We do not generally think that a person's auton-
> omy, or her sense of being able to shape her own
> life, is diminished by the kind of knowledge that

---

[348] Ibid.

[349] Beauchamp, and Childress, 80.

being a delayed identical twin might provide.
Rather, to the extent that personal autonomy and
the possibility of developing one's own life plans
consists in tailoring one's goals to one's given circumstances and endowments, knowledge about
one's limitations and strengths would often seem
to help, rather than hinder, in the fashioning of
autonomous life plans and goals.[350]

Kuhse's view seems to be shared by all the people who today
decide to undergo time-consuming, costly, and sometimes
painful genetic testing to find out if they are carriers of any
genetic disease. Some do so before asking their partner to
commit to them permanently or before trying to conceive offspring. They believe that the information they obtain about
themselves in this way will enable them to make the most autonomous decision possible – both for themselves and for the
person or persons who will be affected by their decision.

All this, namely the generally uncontroversial thesis that
ignorance limits the autonomy of the moral agent, and the corresponding thesis that the pursuit of ignorance about a matter
that concerns us – if knowledge about it is available and offered
to us – means that the person is in such a state that she cannot in
any case be considered autonomous and therefore not the bearer of a right, has led several ethicists to more radical paths: First,
they argue that there is a duty on the part of the moral person
to know her genetic endowment. In particular, they challenge
the theoretical basis presupposed by proponents of the right to
ignorance itself, namely, that moral agents have no moral duty
to know their genetic endowment. Rosamond Rhodes and Ruth
Chadwick, for example, who examine the right to genetic igno-

---

[350] Kuhse, 23.

rance from different perspectives, the first from a deontocratic perspective and the second from a consequentialist perspective, both reach the same conclusion, namely, that the moral agent has an obvious duty to know her genetic constitution and structure, which means that a right to ignorance is inconsistent because if we have a duty to do something, we cannot simultaneously have a right not to do it: The right we have gives us the freedom to do or not to do something, while the duty we have deprives us of the corresponding moral freedom, since it obliges, binds, prevents, or morally restricts us from doing something.[351] Thus, if we grant someone the right to genetic ignorance, they cannot at the same time have a duty to the corresponding knowledge. This is also true in reverse: If we accept the existence of a duty to know our genetic predisposition, it is impossible to accept a right to genetic ignorance at the same time.

Rosamond Rhodes examines the right to genetic ignorance in light of the Kantian tradition. She argues that, contrary to what common understanding and superficial consideration of the subject seem to justify, the autonomy of the moral person imposes on her a duty to genetic knowledge as part of her obligations to her fellow human beings. Specifically, the moral person ought to strive to gain knowledge about her genetic self if she wishes to use that knowledge [a] to contribute to scientific knowledge about the genetic composition of a population group, [b] to expand the available information about the genetic history of one's family, and [c] to discover genetic information about herself and her descendants.[352] According to Rhodes, a moral agent's refusal to obtain genetic information at no particular cost or inconvenience to herself demonstrates a psychological tendency or inclination compa

---

[351] Rhodes, 15.

[352] Ibid., 11.

rable to that of someone who insists to drive her car blindfolded or completely drunk: If her decision had no consequences for others or for herself, there would be no problem. But precisely because driving blindfolded or drunk would cause harm to others or oneself, we consider it the duty of a moral agent not to drive in such a condition. Acknowledging and complying with this duty, according to Rhodes – and also according to common sense – does not limit one's autonomy, but rather strengthens it. The moral person herself could not but freely choose this maxim as a norm of behavior, since only this maxim could become a universal law. The same, Rhodes argues, is true of knowledge of our genetic makeup:

> When I recognize that I am ethically required to be autonomous, I must also see that, since autonomous action requires being informed of what a reasonable person would want to know under the circumstance, I am ethically required to be informed. So, if I have an obligation to learn what I can, when genetic information is likely to make a significant difference in my decisions and when the relevant information is obtainable with reasonable effort, I have no right to remain ignorant. From the recognition of my own autonomy, I have a duty to be informed.[353]

The above gains additional weight when one considers the commitments of the moral agent to others. In particular, in the context of the social relations that individuals develop, they make explicit or implicit commitments to others. When Kant speaks of promises – and any commitment is, at its core,

---

[353] Ibid., 18.

a kind of promise – he insists that it is our perfect duty to others not to make promises that we know in advance we cannot keep, because the contrary maxim would necessarily be self-defeating.[354] In my view, any maxim that would allow one to make a commitment without first making a rudimentary assessment of one's ability to keep it would be equally contrary to the moral agent's perfect duty to the person she is committing. For to undertake something knowing in advance that one cannot fulfill one's obligation is just as contradictory as to undertake something without knowing in advance – or at least having a reasonable suspicion – whether one can fulfill one's obligation: In both cases, such an omission or failure

> would make impossible the promise and the end one might have in making it, since no one would believe that anything has been promised him, but rather would laugh about every such utterance as vain pretense.[355]

By way of illustration, let us consider the case of two persons, one of whom commits herself knowing in advance that she will not be able to keep what she has promised, while the other commits herself without knowing – or having reasonable doubt – that she will be able to keep what she has promised. In the first case, the concept of commitment is void and what Kant describes above occurs. In the second case, any commitment can be kept only under certain circumstances and on a case-by-case basis. In this case, too, the concept of commitment is inconsistent, for its essence is that both the one who

---

[354] Kant, *Groundwork for the Metaphysics of Morals*, 4:442: "Yet I see right away that it [my maxim] could never be valid as a universal law of nature[and still agree with itself, but rather it would necessarily contradict itself."
[355] Ibid., 4:442.

makes it and the one who demands it are convinced that the commitment will be respected except in exceptional circumstances. Reasonable probability, however, presupposes that any commitment is based – at least in the most elementary sense – on knowledge of certain basic facts, otherwise it remains pure speculation.

In the case of our genetic nature, Rhodes argues, circumstances sometimes require more than rudimentary knowledge and describe for the moral agent the duty to know precisely. For example, suppose that two partners planning to have offspring have good reason to believe that they both carry a genetic mutation in the gene HEXA on chromosome 15 that has a high probability of causing their offspring to have Tay-Sachs disease. Both potential parents have cases of Tay-Sachs in their close family, and both belong to populations where the disease is very common (this disease is very common in the Ashkenazi Jewish population). The chance of transmitting Tay-Sachs disease is one in four, and only if both parents are carriers. The disease usually leads to death by age five – sometimes earlier – and by then the child gradually develops visual disturbances, motor clumsiness, mental retardation, and seizures that eventually render her disabled. In such cases, Rhodes argues, parents have a duty to know their own genetic makeup, because to persist in ignorance would be to leave things to chance.[356] The cost of the unfortunate outcome of this peculiar gamble, however, would have to be borne by a child condemned to wait five years for death to be redeemed from a life deprived of all joy and burdened only with untold pain. On the other hand, the knowledge that both parents are carriers of Tay-Sachs disease would probably lead them to another path, possibly adoption, since consciously taking the

---

[356] Rhodes, 18.

risk of giving birth to a child with this disease would mean harming both the child[357] and oneself, which is simply absurd. The same is true for someone who has a reasonable suspicion that she suffers from Huntington's disease and who intends to commit to her partner and start a family. There seems to be an undeniable duty for her, too, to have genetic knowledge and to inform her partner, because only then can she make an informed, autonomous decision.[358] But one also has a duty to one's immediate family to be aware of one's own genetic predisposition, for genetic correlation studies are nowadays a very useful tool available primarily to members of the extended family. Rhodes adds a corresponding duty to society, because research into a genetic disease, especially when the responsible gene varies occasionally, is possible only if individuals make an effort to know their genetic predisposition. In any case, our refusal to know may harm others, and making choices that harm others is by no means a maxim that can be expected or desired to be elevated to the status of a universal law of nature.

Even *possible* harm to others is reason enough for Ruth Chadwick to reject the right to ignorance. But precisely because she is in the tradition of consequentialism, she, unlike Rhodes, does not think it necessary to prove the existence of a duty to know in order to invalidate the alleged right to genetic ignorance. It is sufficient that ignorance causes harm that could easily be prevented if moral agents knew what they were choosing to ignore. Chadwick cannot help but be completely negative concerning the right to ignorance. Chadwick emphasizes that "lack of knowledge can cause harm: decisions made

---

[357] John Harris, *Wonderwoman & Superman: The Ethics of Biotechnology* (Oxford: Oxford University Press, 1992), 79-97.

[358] Jane Wilson, "To Know or not to Know? Genetic Ignorance, Autonomy and Paternalism," *Bioethics* 19, nos. 5-6 (2005): 495.

in ignorance, on matters related to reproduction, for example, can cause harm that could have been avoided."[359]

An important factor in rejecting the right to genetic ignorance, according to Chadwick, is the effect that the possible acceptance of this right would have on social cohesion and the sense of solidarity and responsibility toward others, since the person who invokes the right to genetic ignorance does so for selfish reasons and disregards any responsibility to her immediate or wider social environment, a responsibility that in this case, according to Chadwick, is to participate in genetic mapping and testing programs to identify vital data for her family and the broader population of which she is a part.[360] For example, as I mentioned earlier, Tay-Sachs disease is prevalent in the Ashkenazi Jewish population, apparently due to the practice of extensive inbreeding that was common among this racial group until recently. Tay-Sachs disease is an autosomal recessive mutation of the Hex-A gene on chromosome 15. The fact that the mutation is recessive means that it must be homozygous for the disease to be expressed, i.e., the defective gene must be present at both homologous positions on the chromosome. Precisely because one gene is inherited from the father and the other from the mother, both parents must carry the recessive mutation in their DNA for the disease to be expressed. If, on the other hand, only one of the two is a carrier, the mutated gene cannot be expressed, and the gene already present takes over. In the case of recessive inherited disorders such as Tay-Sachs, genetic screening can reduce or even eliminate the prevalence of the genetic disorder in a given, rela-

---

[359] Ruth Chadwick, "The Philosophy of the Right to Know and the Right Not to Know," in *The Right to Know and the Right not to Know: Genetic Privacy and Responsibility*, eds. Ruth Chadwick, Mairi Levitt, and Darren Shickle, 13-22 (Aldershot: Ashgate, 1997), 18.

[360] Ibid., 20.

tively closed population. It is equally obvious that a person who refuses to participate in genetic screening in such a case, invoking her right to genetic ignorance, may have made that decision only based on selfish reasons, in disregard of her responsibilities to the population group to which she belongs, and in disregard of any sense of solidarity with her fellow human beings. Moreover, the adoption of the right to ignorance could jeopardize the subtle relationship between doctor and patient,[361] since it would call into question the doctor's duty to inform her patient of the possible – in this case genetic – risks and to allow her to choose how to deal with them.[362]

Both the deontological and the consequentialist approaches seem to have difficulties in considering the concepts of *right* and *ignorance* as compatible, at least as far as the possession of information about our genetic endowment is concerned. On the contrary, in their context, knowledge can be more easily presented as a duty for the moral agent. Some philosophers, such as Gilbert Hottois and John Harris, go a step further and consider that the recognition of the right to genetic ignorance, especially when adopted in official normative texts,[363] is reactionary and obscurantist and contradicts both the concept of human rights and morality itself.[364] Within the framework of their argument, if we want to model the language of morality, we can only speak of a *right*, or rather a *duty*, to know, since only knowledge guarantees both autonomy and the promotion of the common good.[365]

---

[361] Andorno, "The Right Not to Know: An Autonomy Based Approach," 436.

[362] Canellopoulou-Bottis.

[363] See Council of Europe, *Explanatory Report to the Convention on Human Rights and Biomedicine* (Strasbourg: Council of Europe, 1997), §67.

[364] Gilbert Hottois, "A Philosophical and Critical Analysis of the European Convention of Bioethics," *Journal of Medicine and Philosophy* 2 (2000): 140.

[365] Harris, and Keywood, 418-419.

So far, I have examined the right to ignorance in general – and not just the right to genetic ignorance – in light of two dominant traditions in the field of moral philosophy, namely Kantian ethics and utilitarian ethics, within which the invocation of the right to ignorance can be seen as self-defeating on the one hand and as either ineffective or harmful on the other. Criticism of the argument considered here, however, is not limited to a review of its theoretical validity, but extends to the way it is applied in the case of cloning. In particular, it has been argued that even if, for the sake of the argument, we could accept the validity of such a right in general – which, as we have seen above, would not be particularly easy – (a) invoking it with respect to cloning would be inappropriate because, even if cloning were applied, it would not – and could not – infringe any right of the clone not to know; (b) even if it did, it would not do so to any greater extent than other morally uncontroversial practices.

Those who argue in this context that cloning violates the clone's so-called right to genetic ignorance hold that (a) if the clone knows her prototype, she will have a real foretaste of her future in its most important aspects, (b) the clone will believe that she knows her future, and (c) the clone's environment, precisely because it is a generally accepted notion that one's genetic makeup determines one's personality and life course, will place certain demands and expectations on the clone.

As for the first thesis about the clone's knowledge of the future, it is now generally accepted that the clone cannot obtain real information about her future by merely observing her prototype, since both the course of a person's life and her personality are only partly determined by her genetic constitution. The environment in which one develops has a much greater influence on one. The clone would naturally develop in a very different environment than her prototype, and therefore her life path and personality would also be different. As for the genetic identity of the clone and the prototype, it should be noted that even in homozygous twins, the only thing they have in common in most cases is their physical appearance – and this to some extent. However, their personalities are always different, and never is the course of their lives identical. The clone as a later twin of a pre-existing (or existing) human would not even have a genome identical to that of her original since she would certainly have emerged from a different egg. It is known that the egg contributes part of the genetic information called mitochondrial DNA.[366] Therefore, the clone and its prototype would in no case be genetically identical, probably not even phenotypically similar, as homozygous twins usually – but not always – are. Thus, the clone's knowledge of her prototype would not give her any real information about her personality and life path, but possibly only the false belief that she has real information about her future.

As for Jonas's thesis that the clone feels – or even believes – that by knowing her prototype she also knows to some extent her personality or future life, this feeling might indeed arise. However, as Dan Brock notes, a person's mistaken belief that she possesses knowledge she does not wish to possess is not a violation of her right to ignorance, since she does not in fact possess that knowledge. To illustrate this, suppose someone mistakenly believes that his car was stolen. The fact that this person believes this to be the case is in no way an actual violation of her property. Even if the clone's social environment were to reinforce her mistaken belief by their behavior toward her, the clone's right to ignorance would not be violated, just

---

[366] Harris, "Goodbye Dolly? The Ethics of Human Cloning," 356; see also n. 18.

as the right to property would not be violated if the social environment of the person who mistakenly believes that her car was stolen were to behave as if it had actually been stolen.[367]

Holm, as we have seen above, admits this difficulty. However, he believes that the fact that the clone herself and those around her believe they know the clone's future is in itself sufficient to impose on the clone a life in the shadow of her prototype and to make cloning so burdensome for the clone that "there are good reasons not to allow it."[368] That both the clone and those around the clone will have the belief that the clone's future is predetermined is not speculation, according to Holm, but a safe conclusion drawn from the observation that genetic determinism is now the dominant interpretation regarding the formation of personality and the development of a person's life, and that this interpretation is extremely unlikely to change in the near future. As long as this observation corresponds to reality, cloning cannot be sufficiently justified morally, since it harms the person directly involved, i.e., the clone. However, I find this argument by Holm unsatisfactory. Precisely because the major premise on which it is based is empirical, the argument retains its validity only to the extent that this premise is assumed to be true. However, the assumption that the majority of people hold the genetic determinism approach is, in my opinion, false – or at least no longer true. For example, the author of this book by no means takes the position that a person's personality, character, and life path are genetically predetermined. I am also sure that many, many people besides me do not share the positions of genetic determinism. So, it would be easy for me to argue that most people reject genetic determinism. But if I did that, I would not be doing much different from what Holm is doing: I

---

[367] Brock, "Human Cloning and Our Sense of Self," 316.
[368] Holm, 162.

would be using a generalization that is impossible to disprove, just as it is, of course, impossible to confirm. For surely no one can examine the thoughts of all people on this question and determine whether or not genetic determinism actually prevails as a tendency. However, if one focuses, as Holm seems to do, on newspaper articles or film productions of the past decade to discern a trend in public opinion on the subject, one might assume that public opinion is indeed influenced by views close to genetic determinism: Nowadays, there are numerous publications on the relationship between the genome and human personality, and the number of films showing clones with a predetermined future and their appeal to the public is constantly increasing. At the same time, of course, anyone who chooses to anticipate the atmosphere surrounding her on the basis of such criteria would also have to assume that liberalism, for example, is blowing its horn and that its replacement is only a matter of time – for there are many more publications on the crisis of liberalism than on the effect of genes on human personality. She should also assume that the average person today believes in magic, given the enormous success of *Harry Potter* and other films series of the kind in recent years. Although all the above criteria do indeed have some value in diagnosing the perceptions of a society, they are not in themselves a reliable means of drawing conclusions. I also believe that the opposite position to Holm's, namely that the majority of people do not share the positions of genetic determinism, has many more arguments in its favor: [a] most religious and philosophical systems defend freedom of the will and one's ability to determine the course of her own life; [b] no reasonable person is suspicious of a criminal's twin brother; [c] human beings generally believe that they themselves can transcend the limits set by nature through the power of their will, etc. And as for Holm's conviction that the dominance of genetic determinism – which he takes as a given – most likely cannot be shaken, I see it is mere speculation. Prevailing beliefs have been known to change, sometimes radically, especially when they are untenable. Helga Kuhse notes, for example, that death has been defined as brain death throughout Europe for decades. In Denmark, however, this definition was not accepted because the public stubbornly clung to outdated biological and other data. Eventually, however, scientific debate and public awareness changed this attitude.[369] Thus, speculation is not a sound criterion for determining the moral value of any decision.

However, even if we accept the validity of the argument about the life in the shadow of her prototype that the clone is supposed to lead, I believe that this argument is not directed against the practice of cloning itself, but against the unprincipled adoption of the positions of genetic determinism by the majority of people today. What schematically underpins the argument about living in the shadow of another is this:

A. Public opinion is full of misconceptions about X.

B. The practice Y falls under X.

C. Practice Y leads to outcome P, which is inevitably burdened by the perception of X.

D. Burdening P with misperceptions about X(Y) unfairly harms, wrongs, and damages P knowingly.

E. It is wrong to knowingly harm, wrong, or damage.

F. Therefore, we should not allow practice Y to produce P.

The above argument, even if we suppose it to consist of true premises, certainly arrives arbitrarily at the conclusion in question, and this because it is only one of the two conclusions

---

[369] Kuhse, 25.

that can be drawn. However, the syllogism does not preclude the other possible conclusion from being drawn. In particular, if the major premise is correct (I have already questioned this above) and if the subsequent minor premises B-E are indisputably correct, the conclusion could also involve the need to change the public's misconceptions about X, and not exclusively our duty to prevent P from occurring. If two inferences can be drawn from a syllogism, the person invoking it must give sufficient reasons why she prefers one inference to the other. In other words, Holm – and the others who argue for the right not to know on the basis of the risk that the clone will spend her life in the shadow of her prototype – would have to present a morally significant case for banning human cloning, and not just informing public opinion (including the clone herself) about the limited validity of genetic determinism instead. Allow me to say that there are insufficient reasons for this particular decision, either in this case or in general. After all, given that human cloning research is subject to an international moratorium and that, even if it were to begin today, it could take several years to reach a level at which humans could be successfully cloned, there would be ample time to inform public opinion of its arbitrary assumptions and to change its attitude toward genetic determinism. Should this succeed – and I see no reason why it should not – the argument for life in the shadow would lose its validity, as the proponents of the argument themselves acknowledge. If we broaden our perspective by going beyond the narrow confines of cloning, we cannot conclude that the argument prevents something new, because usually innovations are treated defensively by public opinion. Let us put in the place of X the complete emancipation of women, a demand made and achieved in the last century. At the beginning of the previous century, a misconception prevailed in public opinion that emancipation would, at best, break family ties. Suffrage clearly falls within the realm of women's emancipation, and certainly early voters struggled with the misconceptions of public opinion. However, this in no way implies [a] that women were wronged, harmed, or damaged by suffrage, [b] that they should be denied the right to vote lest they bear the burden of the misconceptions of public opinion. More generally, as assumed above, basing moral duties or rights on misperceptions of public opinion is highly problematic.[370]

Apart from this, one cannot overlook the fact that all human beings, even though so far no human being has emerged as a clone, sometimes live their lives in the shadow of their ancestors, and that either their ancestors or the descendants themselves, who experience their ancestors' existence as a shadow on their own lives, are responsible for this. In the case of the descendants of the Nazi criminal Hermann Goering, to whom I referred above, the shadow of their ancestor led them to make non-autonomous decisions, as these were more or less based on their mistaken belief that genetic ancestry imposes some sort of predisposition, predicts similarities in personality, etc. Goering was certainly responsible for many despicable things in his life, but certainly not for the misconceptions of his descendants. On the other hand, many ordinary parents, by their own acts or omissions, cast a shadow on their children far heavier than that which the original of a clone could presumably cast on her clone,[371] by undermining their children's sense that they are autonomous subjects, that they are free, and that they have the right to pursue and shape their own future.[372] Still, I do not think anyone would

---

[370] Ibid., 25.

[371] Takala, "The Many Wrongs," 61.

[372] Brock, "Human Cloning and Our Sense of Self," 316.

argue that Hermann Goering should not have offspring even if he himself knew in advance what a shameful course his life would take, and certainly no future parent needs to undergo a psychological examination – or visit a fortune teller – to determine the extent to which she will manipulate her children in the future. So, the danger of the clone living in the shadow of her prototype seems somewhat exaggerated.

Based on the preceding discussion, one might come to the following conclusion: Should human cloning be possible and available as a reproductive method, the clone would indeed possess a kind of knowledge about herself that no one else possesses. Moreover, it is reasonable to assume that both the clone herself and those around her would have knowledge about the clone's personality and life course derived from the personality and life course of her prototype. Neither, however, seems to impose on the clone a life in the shadow of her prototype or to actually harm or injure her. Invoking the risk of imposing a life in the shadow on the clone and consistently asserting the so-called right to genetic ignorance, therefore, do not appear to be morally significant arguments against human reproductive cloning.

V. Keeping one's own future open

Similar to the argument I examined earlier, i.e., the argument that focuses on the clone's supposed right not to know her genetic makeup in order to protect herself from the risk of spending her life in the shadow of her prototype, is the argument that focuses on the clone's right to an open future, the protection of which, its proponents claim, would be anything but certain for the clone, since she would have originated as such. Many believe that the clone, as a more or less identical copy of a pre-existing human being, will be limited in her possibilities, choices, and prospects, since some of these will be closed to her because of her predetermined genetic makeup, a fact that she and her environment will be aware of. Thus, the clone will be deprived of something that all other human beings – who came into existence as a genetic recombination of two different genomes – have: The existence of potentially infinite possibilities and choices, some of which they can freely, spontaneously and autonomously select, and on the basis of which they can construct and pursue an absolutely personal path in life, different from all other corresponding paths. The clone, on the other hand, is constrained in this respect by the given and previously known limits imposed on her by the genome of another human being of whom she is herself the duplicate or copy. Thus, if it is a harm for someone to be limited in her future choices and prospects by another person early in life, in the case of the clone she cannot help but be born already harmed in this respect, since her specific right, that to an open future, was violated long before she was born, namely at the moment of her conception in a laboratory.

Although the right to an open future is one of the most central themes in the cloning debate, it was certainly not coined as a defense for the clones that might exist in the future, but for a very different category of people. For in the early 1990s – when Joel Feinberg first introduced the right to an open future[373] – the progress of genetics toward cloning had not yet reached the point where resorting to subtle moral arguments was necessary or even possible. Instead, Feinberg was concerned with establishing a separate category of rights for children. Specifically, Feinberg distinguishes three categories of rights: (a) those that are common to adults and children (A-C rights), such as the right to bodily integrity; (b)

---

[373] See Feinberg, "The Child's Right to an Open Future."

those that can be granted only to adults (A rights), such as the right to vote; among these he includes a special category he calls autonomy rights, such as the right to free exercise of religion; and (c) those that can be granted primarily to children (C rights).[374] This third category of rights may also apply to adults, but only under certain conditions and in special circumstances. Feinberg further divides this third category into two subcategories: 1. Dependency rights, i.e., rights that arise from the child's dependence on others for the enjoyment of the basic necessities of life – food, shelter, protection. These rights also apply to adults who are unable to care for themselves, and therefore "must, at least in this respect, be treated as children throughout their lives."[375] 2. In *rights in trust*. The latter, according to Feinberg,

> [...] look like adult autonomy rights of class *A*, except that the child cannot very well exercise his free choice until later when he is more fully formed and capable. When sophisticated autonomy rights are attributed to children who are clearly not yet capable of exercising them, their names refer to rights that are to be *saved* for the child until he is an adult, but which can be violated "in advance," so to speak, before the child is even in a position to exercise them. This violating conduct guarantees *now* that when the child is an autonomous adult, certain key options will be already close to him. His right while he is still a child is to have these future options kept open

---

[374] Joel Feinberg, *Freedom and Fulfillment: Philosophical Essays* (Princeton, NJ: Princeton University Press, 1994), 76.

[375] Ibid.

until he is a fully formed, self-determining adult capable of deciding among them. These "anticipatory autonomy rights" in class *C* are […] in effect, autonomy rights in the shape they must assume when held "prematurely" by children. Put very generally, rights-in-trust can be summed up as the single "right to an open future" […].[376]

Against this background, the child's right to an open future seems to be a rather *negative* right,[377] since it imposes an obligation on parents, as well as on the child's wider environment, not to act in such a way as to exclude certain options that are not available to the child *now*, but that can reasonably be expected to be available to her as an adult.[378] The right to procreate, i.e., to decide whether, how, and with which partner to produce offspring, obviously does not concern a child while she is still a child. However, her parents' decision to sterilize her while she is still an infant would deny her the opportunity and right to procreate when she is capable of doing so. Her parents would therefore not be allowed to sterilize her, even if their personal religious or other beliefs compelled them to do so.[379] Similarly, Feinberg argues, suppose a child's parents are Jehovah's Witnesses and therefore reject the possibility of a blood transfusion because of their religious beliefs: They must nevertheless respect their child's right to an open future and allow her to have the blood transfusion if there is a reason

---

[376] Ibid., 76-77.

[377] Miana Lotz, "Feinberg, Mills and the Childs Right to an Open Future," *Journal of Social Philosophy* 37, no. 4 (2006): 538.

[378] Kenneth Henley, "The Authority to Educate," in *Having Children: Philosophical and Legal Reflections on Parenthood*, eds. Onora O'Neill, and William Ruddick, 254-264 (New York: Oxford University Press, 1979).

[379] Dena Davis, "Genetic Dilemmas and the Childs Right to an Open Future,"

to do so. Because otherwise, exercising their right to religious freedom would violate their child's right to an open future, which is even more important in this case because it would deprive her of the ability to make all future choices as an adult, including abandoning her parents' religious beliefs and choosing a different faith.[380] Feinberg, of course, acknowledges that absolute neutrality is not possible in an imperfect world. However, Feinberg believes that neutrality can be achieved to some degree.[381] This requires that parents avoid making serious and irreversible commitments on behalf of their children.[382]

Those who invoke the right to an open future argument in the human cloning debate claim that its application can be justified by a plausible expansion of its scope, since, in their view, serious and irreversible commitments will be made on behalf of clones, such as the selective exclusion of certain future options. In the case of clones, the argument of the right to an open future seems to apply *a fortiori*, since the commitments made on behalf of clones are irrevocable and absolutely irreversible, unlike, for example, in the case of adolescents, where the withdrawal of an option by parents is to some extent reversible.[383] In particular, most of the options that seem to be closed to an adolescent because of the decisions of her parents or her environment can be reopened at any time, either by an unexpected change in the course of her adult life or by her own efforts. For clones, however, there is not even this possibility of recovery, albeit a weak one, since their own future is largely *genetically closed*: The genome, as we know, is generally not affected by the unexpected twists and turns of life, nor by the

---

Hastings Center Report 27, no. 2 (1997): 9.

[380] Feinberg, *Freedom and Fulfillment*, 80-81.

[381] Ibid., 85.

[382] Lotz, 539.

[383] Kuhse, 20.

individual's own efforts. Consequently, the clone can only be created if its right to an open future has already been violated. Thus, since cloning legitimately implies and entails the violation of this right, and since the violation of this right is always morally reprehensible, human reproductive cloning can only be tainted with the corresponding moral wrong, which is *per se* sufficient reason to condemn it morally and consequently to reject it as an option, regardless of any other advantages it may have. After all, as Dworkin argues, rights must take precedence over interests in the event of conflict.[384]

Specifically, opponents of cloning claim that the birth of a clone deprives her of the right to an open future in the following cases: [a] When cloning uses genetic material from a person with severe genetically determined disabilities – for example, serious physical or mental problems – or was otherwise committed to an existence more limited than that of other people. In this case, the clone would not be able to lead a satisfying life. [b] If the genome to be cloned is subjected to pregenetic editing to make certain desirable phenotypic traits predominate over those considered undesirable. In this case, the clone is genetically programmed to strive for and achieve certain things in life that are known to her in advance, while all other possibilities are closed to her in advance. [c] Regardless of [a] and [b], certain future possibilities are closed to the clone in any case, since her genetic material is not the result of a random combination of genes – as in humans by heterologous reproduction – but of the replication of a specific genome. [d] Since the clone will be a copy of an already existing human being, it will create in herself and in her social environment the belief that her future is predetermined, an idea which – regardless of whether it is right or wrong – will in any

---

[384] Dworkin, "Rights as Trumps."

case limit the clone's possibilities and choices and thus deny her the right to an open future.

All this may be true to some extent. But to make a sufficient moral argument against cloning, they must be part of a larger argument. In other words: If we take the position that invoking the right to an open future is in itself a sufficient reason to discredit human reproductive cloning, we must also accept the following: [i] that what we call an open future actually exists, and [ii] that it can be considered a moral right of human beings. Furthermore, we must also accept [iii] that cloning does indeed violate the clone's right to an open future, and [iv] that this fact is so morally problematic that cloning should be morally discredited on this basis. In the context of the above, the objections [a], [b], [c], and [d] fall under premise [iii] of the argument, of which they are a detailed formulation. The weight of the above argument undoubtedly lies in premise [iv], which is its most crucial part: For one could accept the validity of the three preceding premises and still not conclude that the deprivation of the right to an open future is so morally serious as to discredit cloning. In any case, however, in order to arrive at this conclusion, we must accept that the above three conditions are met. However, this cannot be taken for granted.

In particular, the assumption that everyone in general has an open future is often questioned. As we have already mentioned, the character, personality, and life path of each of us are shaped, on the one hand, by our genetic endowment and, on the other hand, by the historical, social and cultural environment in which we emerge. If this is the case – and this view is hardly ever disputed – then it follows that the above factors also limit our future choices by excluding some and leaving others open. In other words, every human being – and not just clones – is born with certain facts about her future already predetermined, and with a certain number of possibilities from which to choose. In any case, however, no one's future is *open* in the literal sense of the term. The future of a child whose mother is HIV-positive, and is also a carrier of HIV from the first moment of her existence, is closed to certain very important future options, as is the future of a child that has been as misfortunate as to be born in civil war-ridden Sierra Leone or in the ghetto of a large city in the Western world. This is not true – at least not to the same extent – for the healthy child of a middle-class European family, although her own future is also by no means completely *open*: It is certainly not open to all the situations and options open to a child born with HIV, or to those of a child born in the middle of a civil war or in a ghetto, nor to all the others denied to her because of her particular genetic makeup and the environment in which she is born and lives. However, it makes absolutely no sense to accuse the parents of children born under these conditions of violating their right to an open future by bringing them into the world.[385] It seems that no one's future is *truly open* anyway, at least not completely so.

Even if we assume that the genome of clones is completely fixed – the role of mitochondrial DNA makes this assumption particularly precarious, as I mentioned earlier – they will not differ significantly in the openness of their future from naturally born children[386] resulting from heterologous reproductive process and subsequent gene combination. Both the former and the latter will be subject to constraints on their future possibilities, constraints imposed on both categories

---

[385] Matteo Mameli, "Reproductive Cloning, Genetic Engineering and the Autonomy of the Child: The Moral Agent and the Open Future," *Journal of Medical Ethics* 33 (2007): 90.

[386] McCarthy, 102.

by exactly the same parameters: By their genome, and their environment. The only difference between clones and natural born offspring is that the former are aware of some of the constraints they face, while non-clones are not. However, non-clones' ignorance of the possibilities their genome denies them in no way guarantees their right to an open future, because such a future is not really offered to them. At best, ignorance of one's limitations merely makes one *feel* that one has an open future. Cloning, then, does not deprive the clone of an open future, any more than heterologous reproduction deprives a non-clone, but of the illusion that there is a new, uncharted territory ahead for them to explore. The future is simply not open to anyone, at least not in the sense in which opponents of cloning seem to perceive it as such. But if there is no open future, then no moral right of clones to it can be assumed, nor the concomitant duty of the rest of us to uphold that right. In the words of G. E. Moore, any moral rule "biding us realize a certain end, can only be justified if it is possible that that end should, at least partially, be realized."[387] In other words, every *ought to* implies that it is true that *it is possible to*, and if it is not possible to, it follows that it is not true that one ought to. In our case, if something cannot be protected – this may be the case for a variety of reasons, most notably the possibility that this something does not exist at all – then it is superfluous to argue for its protection by establishing corresponding rights and duties. Consequently, the major premise [i] of the argument considered here, which assumes that such a thing as an open future actually exists and is offered to humans, must of course be proved if we are to establish the moral right of clones to it, as well as the corresponding moral duties

---

[387] G. E. Moore, *Principia Ethica*, ed. Thomas Baldwin (Cambridge: Cambridge University Press, 1993), §68.

that flow from such a right. However, as can be seen from the above, the assumption of an open future for any human being is anything but valid, and this calls into question the validity of the argument based on the violation of the clone's right to an open future altogether.

But even if for the sake of argument we accept the view that all future possibilities are open to people born through heterologous reproduction, this fact alone does not compel us to assume the existence of a moral right to an open future. Moral rights are established by appeal to moral arguments, not on the basis of what is true in reality at any given time. Otherwise, we would have to recklessly indulge in the naturalistic fallacy and derive moral rights from what actually constitutes reality around us, including wars, diseases, and natural disasters. In other words, for the so-called right to an open future to have a moral basis, it must be shown not only that the possibility of such a future exists, but also that it (a) is due to the moral person, is legitimate, and can be pursued, and (b) can be part of a consistent and meaningful moral agreement. None of these, however, are self-evident; on the contrary, in the case of the right to an open future they are all questionable.

For example, regarding the question of whether and to what extent it is legitimate and desirable for human beings to have an open future, it could be argued that it is not reasonable for anyone to desire a *completely* open future, that is, a future open to *all* possibilities. On the contrary, the entire history of human civilization can be seen as a consistent effort to rule out certain contingencies and pursue other, equally concrete possibilities. Medicine, for example, tries to exclude as much as possible the possibility of disease and premature death, while the education that parents consider their duty to give their children is an attempt to exclude the possibility of them becoming, among other things, criminals, instruments of others, and so on. In other words, many life situations included in the so-called open future of humans – and rightly so, since by definition an *absolutely* open future would include *every possible* life situation – are not considered legitimate and everything is done to prevent them, while others are desired and aspired to. For example, no one would praise parents who send their children to a training camp for terrorists during the summer vacations to keep open the possibility that, should their children fail in some other area, they will at least become skilled terrorists in the future. Similarly, vaccination against hepatitis removes the possibility of minors contracting the virus and makes their futures less open to the life-altering feelings of pain, hope, and despair that any potentially fatal disease brings. However, we do not believe that by shielding the body's defenses in any way, we are jeopardizing one's right to an open future.

With all this I mean that the appeal to the right to an absolutely open future is generally untenable. If open future could be regarded as a right, it would be meaningful only as a right to a future made up of possibilities that a reasonable, mature person would desire to have available, in other words, to a future that is not open to all possibilities, but only to those among whom we wish to be free to choose. Since every right aims to protect a freedom that the moral agent may choose to make use of now, or have available in the future, the right to an open future must refer primarily to the possibilities that the moral person in question wishes to pursue. Thus, it would make sense to speak of a right to an auspicious or hopeful future, i.e., to a future rich in reasonably desirable possibilities (or not intentionally made poorer), but not to an open future without distinction, for no one would reasonably prefer sickness to health or weakness to potency. Invoking the open future as an undifferentiated generalization that does not distinguish between desirable and undesirable futures cannot, therefore, be considered a sound basis for determining the appropriate moral right.

As for the conceptual compatibility of the notion of an open future with that of a moral right, several ethicists question both Feinberg's original approach[388] and the extension of his relevant views to the cloning debate. Focusing exclusively on the second point, we must note that the clone's so-called right to an open future does not seem to be equivalent to other – let me say *more traditional* – moral rights, such as the right to life. On the contrary, the right to an open future – particularly with respect to clones – seems to belong to a category of *nonstandard* moral rights whose arrival on the scene seems to have been somewhat precipitous and, for the most part, not adequately justified, and whose invocation sometimes makes the philosophers who propose them seem, in the eyes of many, like magicians unexpectedly pulling rabbits out of their hats.[389] Of course, the novel ethical problems raised by the rapid advances in biomedicine and genetics require the imaginative redefinition of traditional concepts and, where appropriate, the introduction of new and more functional ones. In the case of the clone's right to an open future, however, it seems necessary to extend the concept of right unnaturally beyond its limits. Consequently, and given the indisputable fact that clones do not exist today, the clone's right to an open future falls, in my opinion, into the broader category of the rights of future generations.[390] How-

[388] See, inter alia, Claudia Mills, "The Child's Right to an Open Future?" *Journal of Social Philosophy* 34, no. 4 (2003): 499-509.

[389] Griffin, 306.

[390] See, inter alia, Robert Elliot, "The Rights of Future People," *Journal of*

ever, the possibility of recognizing such a category of rights is also seen as highly problematic.[391]

In particular, future generations, and in this case clones, do not exist in the present, so there can be no interaction between them and existing humans. This impossibility of interaction, however, makes problematic the notion that clones can have interests *now* and therefore have rights.[392] For how is it possible for "someone else to be wronged, harmed, or damaged" if there is no such 'other' who is wronged by the behavior of a human in the present?[393] According to Ruth Macklin, even the certainty that a person will exist in the future is not a sufficient condition for the recognition of rights *before* that person exists,[394] since the ultimate basis for establishing any moral rights is the self-consciousness of their bearer.[395] Therefore, those who, like clones, do not yet exist but may exist in the future obviously have no such status. Moreover, any recognition of rights for people who do not exist can only be meaningless, since they cannot claim them at present,[396] and it is

---

Applied Philosophy 6, no. 2 (1989): 159-169. On intergenerational justice see, inter alia, John Rawls, *A Theory of Justice* (Oxford: Oxford University Press, 1972), 288-289.

[391] Richard De George, "The Environment, Rights, and Future Generations," in *Responsibilities to Future Generations Environmental Ethics*, ed. Ernest Partridge, 157-166 (New York: Prometheus, 1981), 159.

[392] According to Feinberg, only those with interests can have rights; see Joel Feinberg, "The Rights of Animals and Unborn Generations," in *Ethical Theory: An Anthology*, ed. Russ Shafer-Landau, 409-417 (Oxford: Blackwell Publishing, 2007), 411.

[393] Rahul Kumar, "Who Can Be Wronged?" *Philosophy & Public Affairs* 31, no. 2 (2003): 110.

[394] Ruth Macklin, "Can Future Generations Correctly Be Said to Have Rights?" in *Responsibilities to Future Generations Environmental Ethics*, ed. Ernest Partridge, 151-157 (New York: Prometheus Books, 1981), 152.

[395] Ibid., 153.

[396] Wilfred Beckerman, and Joanna Pasek, *Justice, Posterity and the*

by no means certain that once they exist, they will want to do so. With regard to clones in particular, we cannot even begin to know whether they will consider it their right to be offered an open future. One might assume, of course, that in a future global community made up in part of clones, the hierarchy of values would not be the same and that its members would seek to protect different values by recognizing moral rights in a completely different form, since one of the defining characteristics of humans is their ability to form their own version of what a good life is.[397] In this regard, Bernard Shaw's aphorism is quite astute: "Do not do unto others as you would that they should do unto you. Their tastes may not be the same;"[398] this is even more true for future generations, clones included: Their tastes may be completely different from ours. In other words, future clones may see less value in the existence of potentially infinite future realizations, preferring instead a future that is not as open, but more controllable in advance and thus safer for themselves. In sum, while an open future might be recognized as an accepted right for existing humans if the conceptual content and referents of the concept are expanded accordingly, for future generations, and in this case for clones, this right is particularly difficult to justify because its recognition is by no means self-evident: Its proponents must present morally significant reasons to support their positions in this regard.

As for premise [iii], which assumes that cloning deprives clones of the right to an open future, because,

Environment (Oxford: Oxford University Press, 2001), 22.

[397] Brian Barry, "Sustainability and Intergenerational Justice," in *Fairness and Futurity Essays on Environmental Sustainability and Social Justice*, ed. Andrew Dobson, 93-117 (Oxford: Oxford University Press, 1999), 104.

[398] George Bernard Shaw, *Maxims for Revolutionists* (London: Constable, 2012), 5.

> [a] it may be used the genetic material of a person with
> particularly limited abilities,[399]
> [b] the cloned genome can be genetically modified to
> favor certain phenotypic traits,[400]
> [c] the clone, being a copy of only one genome rather
> than the recombination of two different ones, will be
> deprived of certain future options,[401] and
> [d] the available knowledge about the clone's genome
> will create the belief that the clone's future is predeter-
> mined,[402]

one might note that all these concerns are, on the one hand,
pure speculation – some of them do not even seem plausible
– and, on the other hand, even if we accept their validity, they
do not provide a sufficient basis for assuming that the clone's
right to an open future is actually impaired.

As to the first objection, it would be an unwise decision,
to say the least, to use technology to intentionally create people whom we know in advance will be burdened with certain
inherent problems that will put them at a disadvantage compared to other people and drastically limit their potential and
prospects. This position, however, is not an argument against
cloning on the basis that it violates the clone's right to an open
future, but only against cloning people who are characterized
by particular genetic burdens. In other words, this objection
seems to call for setting limits on human reproductive cloning
rather than showing that cloning as a whole might violate the
clone's right to an open future – regardless of the quality of

---

[399] Mameli, 90.

[400] Davis, 12.

[401] Kuhse, 20.

[402] See Habermas, 103ff.

the cloned genome. At best, it might suggest that the right to an open future is violated only in the case of a particular class of clones, namely those whose genetic material comes from donors whose life is already severely limited. However, it does not seem particularly likely or reasonable that cloning would apply to such cases, and for many good reasons: Our fellow human beings, who for various reasons are sometimes characterized by limited options in their lives, usually have to face and overcome situations that leave no room for thoughts about reproduction in general, and reproductive cloning in particular, since their personal survival is often a daily achievement for them. But even if they could overcome this rather absolute practical limitation, they would certainly be discouraged from trying to produce offspring by cloning, both by the knowledge that they would not be able to raise them and by the desire, common to all human beings, that their offspring should have a better life than the one they themselves have lived.

As for the second possibility of subjecting the genome of the clone to genetic editing to favor the appearance of desirable traits and prevent the appearance of undesirable traits, again this does not seem to be an argument against cloning, but rather against eugenics by means of cloning. Indeed, for eugenics, the production of a desirable genotype and phenotype is the most accurate description of its goals, nature, and mission. However, cloning can be understood *without* eugenics – indeed, it is mainly understood that way today – and eugenics can be understood without cloning, considering that human eugenics already has a long history, while that of human cloning has not even reached its first page. In other words, it is not necessary for eugenics to follow cloning unless we would wish it to. Nor is cloning a kind of eugenics as long as it is not aimed at reproducing a particular phenotype or group of phenotypes, such as the Aryan race. Beyond that, however, we need to seriously discuss whether and to what extent any form of gene reprogramming would violate the clone's right to an open future. For example, gene editing and reprogramming could prevent severe and burdensome phenotypic expressions for the carrier that we now consider sufficient reasons to think that a person's potential is limited. In such a case the future of the clone should probably be considered more open than that of its prototype. In this regard, it is particularly unlikely that a clone whose prototype suffered from Down syndrome, but who does not herself suffer from Down syndrome precisely because the donor's genetic material has been subjected to the appropriate gene editing, would consider that her right to an open future has been violated, since she herself will naturally have many more possibilities than her prototype precisely because she has been genetically reprogrammed.

The third objection, namely, the limitation of the future possibilities of the clone due to the fact that she originated from a single genome and not from a mixture of genes as in heterologous reproduction,[403] suffers, as I have already mentioned, from its scientific basis. This is because, at least in the context of the only potentially functional cloning technique currently available, namely somatic cell nuclear transfer, the genome of the clone will consist of *two* genomes rather than *one*: However small the contribution of mitochondrial DNA – which will be supplied by the oocyte – there will be one. Thus, the future of the clone is in no way predetermined by the life course of its prototype, even in the minds of those who fully accept genetic determinism. Beyond this, however, the example of identical twins shows that this argument also suf-

---

[403] Lori Andrews, "Is There a Right to Clone? Constitutional Challenges on Bans on Human Cloning," *Harvard Journal of Law & Technology* 11 (1998): 655.

fers in its reasoning. In particular, identical twins rarely have an identical life course, they usually form completely different personalities, they even suffer from different diseases, although their DNA is more identical than that of the clone and its prototype: Twins originate from a common ovum and therefore share mitochondrial DNA, which, as I have already noted, will not be the case with clones, since clones originate from a different ovum than their prototype. So, if in homozygous twins the shared genome ultimately determines nothing but their phenotype, why should it be any different in clones? Genetic material seems merely to define a margin for each of us, but one large enough to ensure diversity.[404] According to Ian Wilmut, the creator of Dolly, "[...] genes [...] merely suggest possibilities."[405]

In the case of clones, the predispositions common to their prototypes will define for them a certain range of future options, but a *so broad one* that one can hardly speak of a real exclusion of future possibilities – at least not to any greater extent than in the case of human beings created by other, even natural, methods of reproduction. This is because all humans have certain limits imposed on them by their genome that clearly restrict the openness of their future.[406] However, if the possibility of distinguishing clones from their prototypes is as great as the possibility of distinguishing homozygous twins from each other, then it can hardly be said that clones have a closed future, apart from the fact that each individual can

[404] Michael Tooley, "Moral Status of Cloning Humans," in *Human Cloning*, eds. James F. Humber, and Robert M. Almeder, 65-102 (Totowa, N.J.: Humana Press, 2010), 85.

[405] Ian Wilmut, Keith Campbell, and Cristopher Tudge, *The Second Creation: The Age of Biological Control by the Scientists Who Cloned Dolly* (London: Headline, 2000), 302-303.

[406] Mills, 500.

have only one genome and not another at the same time: If I live in Europe, it is impossible to live in Asia at the same time, but this can hardly be understood as a limitation, because I retain a multitude of options that I cannot exhaust in any case during my lifetime. Each of us is who we are because of our genome and the environment (natural and social) we live in, and in this respect, we cannot be anybody else. If this is true of clones as well, it seems a bit of an exaggeration to claim that cloning violates their right to an open future more than natural reproduction. The fact that clones are forced to make choices within the limits imposed by their genetic structure is not a violation of their right to an open future, since they will still be able to choose among a sufficient number of alternatives.[407] According to Joseph Raz, even the existence of *only two* alternatives – as long as they differ from each other – is a sufficient guarantee of individual freedom.[408]

As for the fourth reason put forward by those who invoke the clone's right to an open future, namely, that the knowledge of her genetic origin produces in her and those around her the belief that her future is predetermined, to the extent that this belief is false, there is, of course, no real violation of the clone's right to an open future. Any infringement that occurs only in the mind of the bearer of the right cannot be considered an *actual* infringement – a right is not infringed merely because the bearer of the right believes that it is: It requires another agent to perform certain acts or omissions for it to be violated. If our mistaken perception that a right is being violated constituted its objective violation, then our mistaken perception that a right is being respected would suffice to establish actual compliance with that right. This is inappropriate, however,

---

[407] Kuhse, 27.

[408] Joseph Raz, *The Morality of Freedom* (Oxford: Clarendon, 1986), 375.

because in this case the judge of whether their right is being violated would be the bearer of the right herself. Thus, if the manner in which the clone was created imposes no greater restrictions on her than those to which other human beings are subjected by virtue of their genetic constitution, and if, consequently, clones, by virtue of their given genome, have the same possibilities of future choices as any other human being – whose genes compel her to be not just anyone but exactly the human being she is – then it is difficult to establish an actual violation of the clone's right to an open future. The clone's belief that her right to an open future is not secured – or has been violated – because of the way the clone was created is not enough to prove actual harm, damage, or injury to that person's interests.

In sum, premise [iii] of the argument, i.e., the one that assumes that cloning actually violates the clone's right to an open future because of the four objections listed and commented above, does not seem to be on solid ground and therefore does not support the argument in question. But strong objections are also raised to the premise [iv] that violating the clone's right to an open future is considered a morally significant reason for discrediting human cloning. Proponents of this argument, then, must first offer some weighty reasons why they believe that the right to an open future is so important that its violation is in itself a sufficient reason to morally condemn cloning as a whole. These reasons, given the form of the argument that revolves around the concept of a right, must lie in the harm that will be done to the clone – or in the injustice that the clone will suffer because of the way she was created. For a negative right, such as that to an open future, cannot be valid in any case for any reason other than if its violation causes harm or injustice in some way to the bearer of that right, which ethics seeks to prevent by recognizing the negative right in question in order to impose the corresponding moral duties on others who might harm the bearer of that right. However, both the notion that the clone is harmed by the deprivation of an open future and the position that the harm to the clone is so great that cloning is morally unjustifiable are highly controversial.

The generally accepted view of harm[409] is that someone is harmed when [a] one, by one's own acts or omissions, usually intentionally and unjustifiably, takes her out of the situation she is currently in – and in which she would prefer to remain – and into a worse situation[410] in which she would not have been, had the other party not intervened[411] – as when one unnecessarily upsets a person who is calming down, just to do so, [b] thwarting an interest of the person concerned,[412] as when we spread false rumors about one in order to hinder her professional advancement, and [c] in a narrower sense, according to Feinberg,[413] when our unjust and unwarranted conduct violates a right of the person concerned and thus hinders an interest of the that person, as when we intimidate someone in order ultimately to prevent her from expressing

---

[409] Bonnie Steinbock, "Wrongful Life and Procreative Decisions," in *Harming Future Persons: Ethics, Genetics and the Nonidentity Problem*, eds. Melinda A. Roberts, and David T. Wasserman, 155-178 (Dordrecht: Springer, 2009), 170.

[410] Herbert L. A. Hart, *Punishment and Responsibility: Essays in the Philosophy of Law* (Oxford: Clarendon, 1970), 214.

[411] Joel Feinberg, "Wrongful Life and the Counterfactual Element in Harming," *Social Philosophy and Policy* 4 (1987): 149.

[412] For Feinberg, interests correspond to *stakes*, in the sense that "a person has a stake in X when he stands to gain or lose depending on the nature or the condition of X." See Joel Feinberg, *Harm to Others* (Oxford: Oxford University Press, 1987), 33ff.

[413] Feinberg, *Harm to Others*, 34.

her opinion.[414] Sometimes we can wrong someone in a third sense, that is, we can unjustifiably violate someone's right but without hurting their interest, such as when we break a promise we made to someone and our breach benefits the other person directly or in the long run.[415] Moreover, obstructing or abrogating someone's interests does not always constitute harm to that person, since it may be justified on the one hand and may involve obstructing interests to which that person was not entitled anyway.[416]

Having said all this, the claim that the clone is harmed by the violation of her right to an open future may be supplemented by [i] the fact that the clone is worse off than in a normal birth because of the way she was created,[417] [ii] that an interest of the clone is unjustifiably thwarted, impeded, or nullified, even though the clone rightfully has that interest; or finally, [iii] that the clone is wronged by our violation of one of her rights, a violation that is burdensome to her because it is not ultimately to her advantage. All these arguments, while they seem perfectly reasonable, cannot, in my view, apply in the case of the clone. This is partly because, many argue, the clone could not have been born in any other way to be in a better situation; partly because no reasonable interest of the clone – on which she can legitimately rely – is unreasonably impaired; and finally, no right of the clone is infringed without any greater benefit to herself. Consequently, the clone can suffer no harm – especially no moral harm – or injustice from being deprived of her right to an open future because she is a copy of an original.

[414] Pietro Denaro, "Moral Harm, Moral Responsibility, Ascriptivism," *Ratio Juris* 25, no. 2 (2012): 152-153.

[415] Feinberg, *Harm to Others*, 35.

[416] Ibid., 35-36.

[417] Strong, "Cloning and Infertility," 280.

The reasons why this is the case can be traced back to the problem of non-identity set forth and analyzed by Derek Parfit.[418] In particular, he argues that anything that is bad must be bad *for someone*.[419] It follows that a decision of ours that is not bad for anyone – in the sense that it does not harm anyone who exists or will exist in the future – cannot be bad in the moral sense of the term.[420] The example that Parfit uses to explore the notion of harm to someone who does not exist is that of a fourteen year old girl who

> [...] chooses to have a child. Because she is so young, she gives her child a bad start in life. Though this will have bad effects throughout this child's life, his life will, predictably, be worth living. If this girl had waited for several years, she would have had a different child, to whom she would have given a better start in life.[421]

The question that naturally arises in this case is whether the fourteen-year-old girl should have waited to ensure better conditions for the child she will give birth to, because the decision to give birth *now* will harm the child that is to be

---

[418] See Derek Parfit, *Reasons and Persons* (Oxford: Clarendon Press, 1987), 357ff. Parfit is not the only one who has been concerned with the possibility of causing harm to people who *are to* exist. For similar analyses, see Michael Bayles, "Harm to the Unconceived," *Philosophy & Public Affairs* 5 (1976): 292-304; Robert M. Adams, "Existence, Self-Interest, and the Problem of Evil," *Noûs* 13 (1979): 53-65; and Gregory Kavka, "The Paradox of Future Individuals," *Philosophy & Public Affairs* 11 (1982): 93-112.

[419] Parfit, 363.

[420] M. A. Roberts, "The Non-identity Fallacy: Harm, Probability and Another Look at Parfit's Depletion Example," *Utilitas* 19, no. 3 (2007): 268.

[421] Parfit, 358.

born.[422] The spontaneous thought of most would be that the girl should wait until she is ready. However, we could give a variety of other reasons for this, but not the viewpoint that the girl's decision to give birth now will harm the child that is to be born. This is because "in the different outcomes, different people would be born. I shall therefore call this the Non-Identity Problem."[423] The Non-Identity Problem consists in the fact that the child that now results from the fertilization of this particular egg will not be the same as the child that later results from the fertilization of another egg, but will be two completely different individuals. The child that the girl wants to have, if not born now, will never be born, because any child born in the future is a different child. Therefore, when this particular child is born, it is particularly difficult to assume that we are causing it harm, that is, that we are imposing on it, through our own actions or omissions, a condition worse than the one it would otherwise have been in, because if we had not brought it into existence, this particular child could not have existed in any other way, either in a better or in a worse condition: If it had not been born now, and in the condition in which it was born, it would never have existed. It seems, then, that there is no child who has been harmed by her mother's decision,[424] since the fact of her birth has not transformed her from a state desirable for herself into an undesirable one, and since no interest of her has been harmed, that is, since no one has caused a negative result of something at stake for the child, by which the child has been harmed.

As far as protecting her rights, for example, her right to a favorable start in life, and in this case, as far as this particu-

---

[422] Jeffrey Reiman, "Being Fair to Future People: The Non-Identity Problem in the Original Position," *Philosophy & Public Affairs* 35, no. 1 (2007): 74.

[423] Parfit, 359.

[424] Kuhse, 26-27.

lar child is concerned, "[...] Even if this child has this right, it could not have been fulfilled. This girl could not have had this child when she was a mature woman,"[425] so she could not preserve her rights. In all of this, of course, there should be some threshold of tolerance so that the problem of non-identity does not legitimize the birth of children who are condemned to suffering from birth, as is the case with children born with Tay-Sachs syndrome, who have a life expectancy of five years and whose entire short lives are condemned to constant suffering. Parfit, like others, sees this limit as a guarantee of a life *worth living*,[426] or at least a *minimally decent* life,[427] that is, a life that cannot be expected to degenerate into "[...] the level of severe disability or incapacity, by virtue of which the child's very existence would constitute for him a net burden and, therefore, an injustice."[428] If this condition is met, it seems problematic to claim that the birth of a child would be detrimental to the child, because if the child had not been born as the person it was born as, it would not have existed at all.[429] In her attempt to clarify Parfit's position, Bonnie Steinbock adds to his working hypothesis two parallel examples, that of Angela and that of Betty, two women who will give birth to their child under circumstances similar to those in Parfit's example:

> Angela is pregnant. Her doctor discovers that she has a condition that will result in mild retardation in her baby. The doctor prescribes a medication that will prevent the retardation. But Angela does

---

[425] Parfit, 364.

[426] Ibid., 358.

[427] Steinbock, 169.

[428] John A. Robertson, *Children of Choice: Freedom and the New Reproductive Technologies* (Princeton, NJ: Princeton University Press, 1994), 122.

[429] Kuhse, 27.

not want to take the medication, because a side effect of the medication is that it can cause mild acne. So she does not take it and as predicted her baby is born mildly retarded. Betty wants to get pregnant. However, she is on medication that has the following side effect: if she gets pregnant while on medication, her baby will be born mildly retarded. Going off the medication is not a feasible option, as it would aversely affect her health as well as her fertility. Fortunately, she only needs to take the medication for a few months. Her doctor advises her to wait to get pregnant until she is off the medication. But Betty does not want to wait. She plans to visit her family during her summer vacation, and so she wants to have the baby in June at the latest. She gets pregnant right away and has a baby in June who, as predicted, is born mildly retarded.[430]

According to Steinbock's view, Angela actually harms her child because she arranges things as to have it born in a more difficult situation than the one in which *the same* child would have been born if the mother had acted differently. Betty, on the other hand, did not harm the child she gave birth to, because she could not have given birth to the same child if she had waited a few months to complete her treatment.

As for cloning, the case seems to be exactly the same. For even if we assume that the individuals from whom the genetic material to produce the clone is derived are fertile, and therefore the clone could have been conceived naturally as a non-clone, it would not be the same individual even if a somatic cell

---

[430] Steinbock, 169-170.

nucleus from the male donor and an egg cell from the female donor were used in cloning, since the recombination of the genetic material occurs at conception and not during cloning.[431] Even if the clone in question – simply because she would have been born as such – were to suffer impairments that those who originated as non-clones do not have to suffer, we could not assume that she was harmed or wronged by her parents. This is because the conditions she will experience will be the only one possible for her, and not the worst possible among the probable conditions, into which she would have fallen because of the actions or omissions of her ancestors – assuming, of course, that her life would not otherwise have been fraught with serious problems, so that the very fact that she came into being would be a burden to the clone.[432] As Ruth Macklin notes, if we argued otherwise, we would have to assume that if the clone had never existed, it would be in a better situation than the one she is in because she exists as a clone. This position could be formulated in the context of a metaphysical hypothesis, but not as a moral argument, since this position presupposes and requires a comparison between existence and nonexistence, and ultimately leads to a preference for the latter.[433] This is absurd, however, since what is compared here is something that is known to us, that is, existence, and something we completely ignore, that is, non-existence. Even at this level, however, the position that it would have been better if the clone had not existed does not seem coherent, as Elizabeth Harman notes:

> Either he is better off than he would otherwise have
> been (because life can be compared to non-exis-

---

[431] Justine Burley, and John Harris, "Human Cloning and Child Welfare," *Journal of Medical Ethics* 25 (1999): 109.

[432] Kuhse, 27.

[433] Macklin, "Splitting Embryos on the Slippery Slope," 219.

tence, and it is better to have a life worth living than not to exist), or he is not worse off because he is neither worse off nor better off (because existence cannot be compared to non-existence). Either way, he is not worse off than he would have been had she not performed that action [...] Furthermore, it seems that the only candidate explanation of her action's wrongness is that it harms; so it seems her action is not wrong.[434]

According to Helga Kuhse, the view that cloning constitutes harm to the clone because it affects her rights – including the right to an open future – requires the adoption of a non-person-affecting view of the concept of harm or, in other words, a *same-number* but not a *same-person* view.[435] According to this view, harm does not concern *one and the same* person, because a person cannot be harmed if that person could not possibly have existed other than as she exists, but two different possible persons between which we can choose which of them exists and which does not. According to Parfit, this approach, which he calls claim 'Q,' provides a solution to the problem of non-identity and is formulated as follows:

> If in either of two possible outcomes the same number of people would ever live, it will be worse if those who live are worse off, or have a lower quality of life, than those who would have lived.[436]

---

[434] Elizabeth Harman, "Harming as Causing Harm," in *Harming Future Persons: Ethics, Genetics and the Nonidentity Problem*, eds. Melinda A. Roberts, and David T. Wasserman, 136-154 (Dordrecht: Springer, 2009), 138.

[435] Kuhse, 27.

[436] Parfit, 369.

This change in the perspective from which harm is perceived allows for the ethical discrediting of reproductive practices such as cloning when the human beings produced have a significantly worse quality of life than the same number of different human beings that could be produced by other means. Returning to Parfit's example, that of the fourteen-year-old girl contemplating whether or not to have her child, if the girl ultimately decides to give birth to the child she is carrying, she has caused non-personal harm, because if she had waited, she could have given birth to another child under better circumstances. Parfit's notion of harm is adopted by several modern thinkers to address issues of reproduction more broadly. Allen Buchanan and Dan Brock, building on Parfit's Q claim, formulate their own axiom, the N principle:

> Individuals are morally required not to let any child or other dependent person for whose welfare they are responsible experience serious suffering or limited opportunity or serious loss of happiness or good, if they can act so that, without affecting the number of persons who will exist and without imposing substantial burdens or costs or loss on themselves and others, no child or other dependent person for whose welfare they are responsible will experience serious suffering or limited opportunity or serious loss of happiness or good.[437]

---

[437] The so-called Principle N, which was originally formulated by Brock. See Dan Brock, "The Non-Identity Problem and Genetic Harms – The Case of Wrongful Handicaps," *Bioethics* 9, nos. 3-4 (1995): 273. For a more developed version of this see also Buchanan, Brock, Daniels, and Wikler, 249. The quote is from the second.

The above concept would possibly allow the birth of a person by cloning to be considered a harm – though not a harm to a particular person – because this would necessarily entail the loss of the clone's right to an open future, since if another person had been born as a non-clone instead of the clone, that person would not suffer from this restriction. This would require, however, that one adopts a non-personal conception of harm that does not seem entirely convincing to many, including me. And even if one were willing to adopt the above concept, it would have limited application to cloning. In particular, the claim that cloning, unlike other methods of reproduction, deprives the clone of the right to an open future and therefore should not be used would carry weight only in the case of a couple who could have conceived offspring using other methods of reproduction but who chose cloning for their own reasons. In the case of couples who cannot produce offspring by other means, the requirement to create the same number of individuals that both Claim Q and Axiom N impose is not met, since these couples will either produce offspring by cloning or have no offspring at all. Moreover, in the case of individuals who view cloning as the only way to prevent the transmission to their children of a genetic disease of which they are carriers, the condition of preventing 'significant harm to themselves and others' under claim N is not satisfied, nor is preventing the possibility that the children who are eventually born will have 'a lower quality of life than those who would have lived.' In light of the fact that cloning, for many reasons, some of which I have already mentioned, as a right to reproductive freedom is primarily and mainly meaningful in the case of infertile couples – or individuals – and for those who do not want to risk passing on an inherited genetic disease to their offspring, it seems that even the non-personal harm view cannot convince us that partially and insignificantly limiting for the clone of one of her rights is so morally significant that cloning should not be considered a morally legitimate reproductive option.[438] In sum, the position that cloning harms the clone because it violates the clone's right to an open future, and therefore cannot be morally justified as a reproductive method, cannot be based on neither the personal nor the non-personal view of harm. However, if no harm or injustice can be done to the clone by creating it as such, it is difficult to accept that a right – in this case, the right to an open future – is violated, unless we are willing to accept that the violation of a right means no harm to the bearer of that right – which, however, makes no sense, at least in my opinion.

Finally, the claim that clones are deprived of their right to an open future, one that, on the contrary, others enjoy, and that this alone is sufficient to suppose that clones are so harmed by the mere fact that they have come into existence, that it would have been better for themselves if they had not existed at all, seems to unduly expand the range of reasons for which we think that life can be a burden to a human being and, accordingly, to make the notion of a dignified or worth-living life extremely narrow. This restriction, however, can only exclude from procreation a number of our fellow human beings whose offspring we nevertheless believe could live a reasonably worth living life. If we assume that the alleged deprivation of the clone's right to an open future is a reason not to create clones, we should assume the same – and even more so – for the cases of people who, for genetic reasons, are to be born, for

---

[438] Kuhse, 29.

example, deaf-mute or mildly mentally retarded. We should assume the same for the heir to the throne of a royal house, argues John Harris.[439] The future of the heir to the throne is largely determined by the demands of the subjects or citizens of the nation she is to rule by virtue of her ancestry. However, the fact that the future of the heir to the throne in question is much more closed than that of other people does not force us to assume that her royal parents are doing something morally indefensible when they choose to procreate.[440] In the case of procreation, Steinbock argues, the bar must be set at the level of a minimally decent or worth-living life, but no higher,[441] since life itself can be sufficiently satisfying for its bearer, regardless of the constraints that distinguish it in any particular case.[442]After all, as I have already shown, the creation of twins, whether by nature or by cloning, can by no means considered an injustice to them.[443]

---

[439] John Harris, *On Cloning* (London: Routledge, 2004), 89.

[440] Mameli, 92.

[441] Steinbock, 169.

[442] John A. Robertson, "Involuntary Euthanasia of Defective Newborns: A Legal Analysis," *Stanford Law Review* 27, no. 2 (1975): 254.

[443] Robertson, "The Question of Human Cloning," 10.

3. Non-conclusive Postscript

Hundreds of pages to reach no firm conclusion may seem like a big waste of time. But this is usually the case with ethics and philosophy in general, so please do not make any higher claims: Especially with ethics, one cannot wish for more than tentative conclusions; if this were not the case, there would not be different moral traditions, but only one that would have prevailed. Nor would all moral debates still be open and active.

That being said, however, the journey has been anything but barren. This book may not have reached solid conclusions about whether and how human reproductive cloning affects our moral status – a status we readily ascribe to ourselves, and probably for good reason – as unique individuals who possess that peculiar and elusive quality, *dignity*; nonetheless, I believe that discussions such as these allow us to deepen our own insight, and I wish that had been the case with this book.

My primary goal was to explore whether and to what extent the moral legitimization and consequent legalization of human reproductive cloning would compromise the uniqueness of the clone or the prototype and diminish the dignity of both, as well as the concept of human dignity as a whole. Following Antisthenes' view that "wisdom begins with the examination of the meanings," I have set out first to examine the key concepts in this debate, namely human uniqueness and human dignity, while of course also attempting to provide a broad overview of cloning in general, focusing on somatic cell nuclear transfer in the context of human reproductive cloning.

The discussion of these two key concepts, uniqueness and dignity, was not at all enlightening for me, but rather reinforced in me the confusion that surrounds these two concepts anyway: I could not see why the human species is unique in a way that other species are not, nor in what sense individual humans are unique such that they are different in this respect from every other individual human being, as well as from every other being, living or not; nor could I see what human dignity consists of, such that it is unique to humans.

As for uniqueness, I have postulated that both qualitative and quantitative uniqueness apply to every single instance of nature, not just humans, and that this is both an empirical conclusion and a logical imperative, as McTaggart's law of the dissimilarity of the diverse shows. In light of this, what we mean when we say that the human species is unique is probably not that it is distinct from all other species, while at the same time each individual human being is unique because it is distinct from all other individual human beings and also from every other individual instance of nature; rather, by uniqueness we mean *superiority*. Human beings are superior to other beings in that they are *persons* in contrast to every other *instance of nature*. On the question of what makes a person a person, I have focused on four possible answers among many others (some I have omitted, e.g., possessing a soul), namely, rationality, self-consciousness, agency, and incommunicability: In my view, these are the concepts most closely related to the subject of this book, human reproductive cloning. But again, I have not understood why only humans can be considered unique in the sense I have described, since several other beings are at least to some extent rational, have self-consciousness, act for and toward ends, and are also in some sense incommunicable – not, of course, in the sense in which Crosby understands the concept. Nevertheless, it might occur to us that while all these four capacities alone are not sufficient to establish human uniqueness, they could very well serve as the basis for something that is indeed unique to humans: Namely, that although other individual beings may also possess these capacities, in humans these capacities have somehow become the basis of a *further fact*. This further fact is often and by many considered to be what we call human dignity, a concept that is as conceptually elusive as uniqueness – if not more so. As the most convenient way to arrive at the concept of dignity, I have chosen the concept of incommunicability, but I know that there are many alternative paths to this concept. To these I must add that in order to keep the debate about human reproductive cloning open, I believe that it is necessary to move from uniqueness to some relevant concept, and dignity is probably the best candidate for this. This is because human reproductive cloning seems to pose no threat whatsoever to human uniqueness from any conceivable point of view: Since human reproductive cloning aims to create new human beings, it cannot be proven empirically or logically that these new human beings would not be as unique as their prototypes are. In any case, many understand human uniqueness as overlapping with human dignity to a great extent, and the belief is deeply rooted that human uniqueness is either conceptually identical to human dignity or that human dignity derives from human uniqueness.

Regarding dignity, I thought it more appropriate for the subject of this book to follow Crosby's train of thought and examine the concept of dignity through the notion of incommunicability. Crosby's line of reasoning is quite simple: All living beings are unique in some sense, in that they are incommunicable, at least to some degree: They all possess an *inner center* that becomes richer and deeper as we move up the scale of existence. At the top of the scale is the human being, whose inner center, with its richness and depth, constitutes the *infinite abyss of its existence*, and this is what makes the selfhood of the human person infinitely incommunicable, that is, existing *as if the others did not exist*. It is in this infinite, incommunicable selfhood of the human person that dignity seems to be rooted. Crosby's line of thought, at least in my opinion, seems to capture the meaning of the term in such a way that it encapsulates all the major views on dignity from Seneca to Immanuel Kant. Crosby's 'infinite abyss of the inner center' is the ground for 'dignitas' as it appears in Seneca, and for 'Würde,' that is, inner worth, in Kant. In each case, human beings are distinguished by the fact that they admit 'of no equivalent' and are hence 'exalted above any price' because they possess that ineffable, incommunicable self that gives them dignity, a quality that distinguishes the species as a whole, but also each individual member of it, and which enables each of us to stand out from our fellow humans, but also from the rest of the creation. This makes it necessary to distinguish between two kinds of dignity, *generic* or *impersonal* dignity and *personal* dignity, the latter being either a 'constellation of moral rights,' or the word for a very specific moral status. Accordingly, human persons have genuine merit, i.e., dignity, while everything else can only have a price. In both respects, dignity seems to play a role in the debate about human reproductive cloning, either directly or indirectly: It may concern the idea of human dignity as such, i.e., the special moral status we ascribe only to human beings, or the dignity of individual human persons. I have argued that, in my view, human reproductive cloning does not seem to affect human dignity in its impersonal sense in any way. In terms of dignity in the personal sense, admitting human reproductive cloning is only likely that it might affect some among this constellation or rights that support dignity, but not dignity as an indicator of moral status. Thus, if concerns about human dignity were to enter the moral debate about human reproductive cloning, it could only be because some applications or manifestations of cloning would violate certain moral rights that are based on dignity. To this end, I have focused on five rights that seem to me to be particularly relevant to the debate, in the sense that the moral acceptance and subsequent legalization of human reproductive cloning could be seen as either a sufficient or necessary condition, or both, for the promotion or violation of these rights and thus of human dignity.

I first examined two arguments that seem to support the view that human reproductive cloning promotes and enhances human dignity: The right to science and the right to reproductive freedom. Regarding the first argument, it is often argued that a ban on cloning would impede research by blocking certain avenues for researchers and thereby diminishing the overall potential of scientific research in genetics. Thus, if there is such a right, and if respecting that right means allowing human reproductive cloning, then any ban on cloning would be a violation of that right and thus of human dignity vis-à-vis researchers. I have argued that while there are good reasons to accept the right to science as either a moral right or a human right, if human reproductive cloning is understood as I believe it should be, that is, the creation of new human beings identical to existing ones, i.e., clones, then there are no good reasons to believe that it depends on the actual performance of human reproductive cloning. To assume otherwise would be to argue that not allowing actual nuclear testing in the real world diminishes the potential in the field of nuclear fission and that this violates human dignity vis-à-vis researchers, so nuclear testing should be allowed for the sake of preserving dignity, which would be quite absurd. On the contrary, it is almost a commonplace that there is not only one way that leads to the development of science and research. But even if there were no other paths than this one, the progress of science cannot be an end in itself and thus justify everything: Joseph Mengele might have chosen such a line of defense for his despicable experiments on human beings, and I think I need add nothing more to prove my point.

When it comes to reproductive freedom, things are not so simple. For some people, reproductive cloning may be the only chance they have to produce biologically related offspring. This is true not only for same-sex couples or individuals, but also for people who carry risky genetic mutations that in some cases even preclude the possibility of having children. Although this view is plausible, I do not believe that it necessarily leads to moral acceptance of human reproductive cloning as a means of preserving the right to reproductive freedom. The reason is that the right to reproductive freedom is by its nature a negative right. That is, its primary goal is to neutralize all possible threats to the possibilities offered to moral agents in exercising their right to reproduce in the here and now, but it does not in any way aim to ever create new possibilities – and, of course, reproductive cloning is not yet a possibility offered to moral agents in the here and now; at best, it may be offered sometime in the relatively near future, and not without considerable effort on the part of scientists. Negative rights, however, compel us to refrain from certain acts so that the bearers of those rights can freely exercise them, but they by no means compel us to perform certain acts so that those rights can be exercised. In particular, the right to reproductive freedom is intended to protect the freedom to choose with whom to have children, how many, and at what intervals. However, this freedom of choice presupposes possibilities that are already available – the right to reproductive freedom does not require us to *create these possibilities from scratch* or to supplement them with new ones. Thus, while expanding people's reproductive freedom might be *a good reason* to morally accept and legalize human reproductive cloning, banning cloning as a morally or legally defensible option does not seem to violate the dignity of those people, just as, had in vitro fertilization not evolved into a safe and affordable reproductive method, no one's dignity would have been violated.

The argument that focuses on the genomic uniqueness of the clone and prototype, which will inevitably be lost forever for clones and their prototypes if human reproductive cloning is legitimized, seems to overlook crucial scientific evidence and therefore fails to convince, at least not me: The explanations provided by science are convincing enough to prove why this can never be the case – the contribution of mitochondrial DNA in shaping our genome, as well as the fact that genes do not remain stable during pregnancy but are subject to constant mutations, as random factors and the peculiarities of each prenatal environment make it arbitrary which of the genes present are expressed and which are not, make genomic identity absolutely impossible. However, the same is not true for phenotypic identity or similarity, which is very close to identity: It is more than likely that clones are indeed phenotypically identical to their prototypes, or at least strikingly similar to them, and this would presumably be a great burden on both the clones and the prototypes, either because they will believe that they are identical in general and not just in appearance, or because they will be treated as such by the others. To find an answer to the question of how severe such a burden might be for the clones and the prototypes, we have no choice but to turn to the naturally produced identical twins that already exist: As John Harris aptly notes, with respect to phenotypic identity, 'artificial clones raise no difficulty which is not already raised by the phenomenon of natural twins.' For my part, I know of no strong moral argument against twin pregnancy, nor could I imagine one, try as I might. The third point of the argument based on uniqueness, that the clones and the prototypes have the same character traits and could be identical in this respect, is based entirely on genetic determinism, which to my knowledge has not yet been proven either empirically or scientifically: Both common knowledge and scientific evidence show that our character is shaped in part by our genetic makeup and in part by the environment in which we live. And even if it were possible (we have seen that it is not) to create two identical genomes, it remains absolutely impossible to create two identical environments, especially if they are years or decades apart. All in all, the argument that the loss of genomic, phenotypic or character uniqueness (or all three) is inevitable, is for me a very weak argument based on misconceptions and insufficient scientific knowledge.

The most philosophically challenging argument against human reproductive cloning is, in my opinion, the one that focuses on the right not to know one's own genetic makeup. This right would be severely violated in the case of clones, since they would be forced to have genetic knowledge about themselves that is not available to naturally born humans. I will leave aside all objections to the question of whether such knowledge is inevitable or can be prevented, and confine myself only to the general idea of the right not to know. At the very outset I must say that a general right not to know is for me the epitome of a *contradiction in terms*. Perhaps it is the Kantian in me who says this, but I also cannot see how not knowing one's genetic makeup could be a sign of personal virtue or would maximize pleasure; that is, a general right not to know could, in my view, only be in conflict with all three major traditions of ethics, virtue ethics, consequentialist ethics, and deontological ethics. As for the latter tradition in particular, and especially its most dominant version, Kantian ethics, ignorance can only be seen as a *curse*, but never as a condition worthy of the protection and status of a *moral right*: Ignorance in general can only be a limitation on the autonomy of the moral agent, and therefore the maxim that leads to self-imposed ignorance could never be elevated to the status of a universal law. It is true that moral agents – me included – tend from time to time to deliberately remain ignorant of certain details that are available to them about their physical condition, their life expectancy, and so on. But *inclination* is no reason to establish universal laws: These must be approved by reason in the first place, so that they are compelling for all. In Kant's view, inclination and impulse constitute what he calls 'alien causes,' while the freedom of the will must be 'a causality in accordance with unchangeable laws' in order to be 'autonomy, viz. constitute the property of the will to be a law unto itself,' and this 'denotes only the principle of acting according to no other maxim than that which can also have itself as a universal law as its object.' The question, then, is: Could the maxim 'noli sapere' be elevated to the status of a universal law, instead of its opposite 'sapere aude'? As we have already seen, Kant himself gives an emphatic answer to this question in *What is Enlightenment?* Against this background, the fact that one does not actually want to know details about one's genetic makeup may indicate an impulsive reaction to the possibility of learning something distressing or sad about oneself, but not an intention to act according to a maxim that one believes can serve as a universal law. I remain skeptical about whether ignorance *in general* can be considered a moral right, nor am I convinced that this could be the case *in certain circumstances*: To return to the clone, who would presumably be burdened by unwanted knowledge about his genetic make-up, genetic predispositions, limitations, etc., I can also see a much more compelling *duty to know*, because knowledge of all these things, however burdensome, would enable the clone to avoid risks, to turn to a more promising lifestyle, to inform others about her genetic particularities when circumstances require her to disclose such information, as is the case with Tay-Sachs syndrome, and so on. To conclude, even though the right to genetic ignorance seems meaningful from a legal point of view, given the rapid developments in genetics and the fact that genetic information may not be provided against one's will, it is still not, in my opinion, a strong argument against human reproductive cloning.

The same applies to the argument invoking the violation of the clone's right to an open future. On the one hand, it is questionable whether and to what extent there is such a thing as an *open future* anyway, since it seems that fate and decisions made by persons other than the person concerned, usually parents, largely determine the future even of naturally born children. On the other hand, especially in light of the discussion of the weaknesses of genetic determinism, it is quite doubtful that being born a clone would seriously limit one's ability to develop freely and 'at random.' In other words, the creation of a clone does not seem to me to limit a person's future in ways sterilization in childhood or the refusal of a blood transfusion would – and it was precisely such cases that Joel Feinberg was aiming at when he introduced the right to an open future. Moreover, if every single clone could be born either as a clone or not at all, the question of a 'not-so-open future' as opposed to no future at all arises: If violating the right to an open future harms someone, then there seems to be no harm to clones in this case, unless bringing one into existence in the only way this could be possible can be considered a harm. But one can always argue that while cloning does not harm clones by limiting their future in significant ways, the human beings produced would have a significantly worse quality of life than the same number of different human beings that could be produced by other means – this is what Parfit calls *impersonal harm*. I really cannot see why the same number of humans would have a significantly better life if they were born as non-clones. This would have to be proven beyond a reasonable doubt by pointing to specific significant disadvantages that clones would have compared to non-clones, and so far, I cannot name any. Furthermore, the claim that cloning, unlike other methods of reproduction, deprives the clone of the right to an open future and therefore should not be used, would only be valid if the couple considering cloning as an option were a couple who could have produced offspring using other methods of reproduction but chose cloning for their own reasons. In the case of couples who cannot produce offspring by other means, the requirement to produce the same number of individuals that both Claim Q and Axiom N impose is not satisfied, since these couples will either produce offspring by cloning or have no offspring at all. Moreover, in the case of individuals who view cloning as the only way to prevent the transmission to their children of genetic diseases of which they are carriers, the condition of preventing 'significant harm to themselves and others' under claim N is not satisfied, nor is preventing the possibility that the children who are eventually born will have 'a lower quality of life than those who would have lived.' Given the fact that cloning, for many reasons, some of which I have already mentioned, is mainly advocated as a right to reproductive freedom for infertile couples – or individuals – and for those who do not want to risk passing on an inherited genetic disease to their offspring, it seems that even the non-personal harm view does not suffice to convince us that cloning should not be considered a morally legitimate reproductive option.

All in all, it seems to me so far that human reproductive cloning can neither promote nor violate the uniqueness of human beings, their dignity, or certain rights based on – or, deriving directly from – human dignity. I have been unable to find any evidence that human reproductive cloning is in principle detrimental to the moral status of human beings or diminishes the value or values normally accorded to them. In this sense, human reproductive cloning can only be *morally neutral*, at least in my view. This is not to say, of course, that I have exhaustively discussed the issues addressed here, nor that the debate over human reproductive cloning should be limited to principles and values: Not infrequently, perspectives that may be morally defensible in theory turn out to be disastrous in practice. The production of 'identical' human copies is the pinnacle of our science, imagination, and possibilities to date, and when it comes to iconic achievements such as these, there must always be a 'caute!' alongside Kant's 'sapere aude.' That said, I am inclined to believe that the moral debate over human reproductive cloning would be more appropriately – and much more fruitfully – conducted if it focused more on the likely consequences of cloning and less on principles and values.

References

Adams, Robert M. "Existence, Self-Interest, and the Problem of Evil." *Noûs* 13 (1979): 53-65.

Ahlberg, Jaime, and Harry Brighouse. "An Argument Against Cloning." *Canadian Journal of Philosophy* 40, no. 4 (2010): 539-566.

Allison, Henry. *Kant's Groundwork for the Metaphysics of Morals: A Commentary*. Oxford: Oxford University Press, 2011.

Andorno, Roberto. "The Right not to Know Does not Apply to HIV Testing." *Journal of Medical Ethics* 42, no. 2 (2016): 104-105.

Andorno, Roberto. "The Right Not to Know: An Autonomy Based Approach." *Journal of Medical Ethics* 30, no. 5 (2004): 435-440.

Andrews, Lori. "Is There a Right to Clone? Constitutional Challenges on Bans on Human Cloning." *Harvard Journal of Law & Technology* 11 (1998): 644-681.

Annas, George. "Human Cloning." *American Bar Association Journal* 83 (1997): 80-81.

Antisthenis. *Fragmenta*. Edited by Fernanda Decleva Caizzi. Milano, and Varese: Instituto Editoriale Cisalpino, 1965.

Aquinas, Thomas. *Summa Theologica* (Notre Dame, IN: Christian Classics, 1981).

Aristotle. *Metaphysics*. Translated by Hugh Tredennick. Cambridge, MA: Harvard University Press, 1989.

Bailey, Ronald. "Human Cloning Experiments Should Be Allowed." In *Cloning*, edited by Paul Winters, 73-77. San Diego, CA: Greenhaven Press, 1998.

Barglow, Raymond. "Therapeutic Cloning Can Save Lives." In *The Ethics of Human Cloning*, edited by John Woodward, 30-36. Farmington Hills, MI: Thomson Gale, 2005.

Barry, Brian. "Sustainability and Intergenerational Justice." In *Fairness and Futurity Essays on Environmental Sustainability and Social Justice*, edited by Andrew Dobson, 93-117. Oxford: Oxford University Press, 1999.

Bayles, Michael. "Harm to the Unconceived." *Philosophy & Public Affairs* 5 (1976): 292-304.

Baylis, Françoise. "Human Cloning: Three Mistakes and an Alternative." *Journal of Medicine and Philosophy* 27, no. 3 (2002): 319-337.

Beauchamp, Tom L., and James F. Childress. *Principles of Biomedical Ethics*. Oxford University Press, Oxford, 1979.

Beckerman, Wilfred, and Joanna Pasek. *Justice, Posterity and the Environment*. Oxford: Oxford University Press, 2001.

Beecher, Henry. "Ethics and Clinical Research." *New England Journal of Medicine* 274, no. 24 (1966): 1354-1360.

Beitz, Charles R. "Human Rights as a Common Concern." *American Political Science Review* 95, no. 2 (2001): 269-282.

Bellomo, Michael. *The Stem Cell Divide: The Facts, the Fiction, And the Fear Driving the Greatest Scientific, Political and Religious Debate of Our Time*. New York: AMACOM, 2006.

Benn, Stanley I. "Abortion, Infanticide and Respect for Persons." In *The Problem of Abortion*, edited by Joel Feinberg, 92-104. Belmont, CA: Wadsworth Publishing Company, 1973.

Bezanson, Randall P. "Solomon Would Weep: A Comment on In the Matter of Baby M and the Limits of Judicial Authority." *The Journal of Law, Medicine & Ethics* 16, nos. 1-2 (1988): 126-130.

Biesecker, Barbara B. "Goals of Genetic Counseling." *Clinical Genetics* 60 (2001): 323-330.

Birnbacher, Dieter. "Copying and the Limits of Substitutability." In *The Aesthetics of and Ethics of Copying*, edited by Darren Hudson Hick, and Reinold Schmücker, 3-18. London: Bloomsbury Academic, 2016.

Birnbacher, Dieter. "Human Cloning and Human Dignity." *Reproductive BioMedicine Online* 10, Supplement 1 (2005): 50-55.

Boethius. "Treatise against Eutyches and Nestorius." In *The Theological Tractates*, translated by H. F. Stewart, and E. K. Randch. London: W. Heinemann, 1918.

Bostrom, Nick, and Eliezer Yudkowsky. "The Ethics of Artificial Intelligence." In *The Cambridge Handbook of Artificial Intelligence*, edited by Keith Frankish, and William M. Ramsey, 316-334. Cambridge: Cambridge University Press, 2014.

Brendan, Tobin, Chamundeeswari Kuppuswamy, Darryl Macer, and Mihaela Serbulea. *Is Human Reproductive Cloning Inevitable: Future Options for UN Governance*. Yokohama: United States University – Institute for Advanced Studies, 1997.

Broad, C. D. "McTaggart's Principle of the Dissimilarity of the Diverse." *Proceedings of the Aristotelian Society*, *New Series* 32 (1931-1932): 41-52.

Brock, Dan. "Cloning Human Beings: An Assessment of the Ethical Issues Pro and Con." In *Clones and Clones: Facts and Fantasies about Human Cloning*, edited by Martha Nussbaum, and Cass R. Sunstein, 141-164. New York: W. W. Norton Co., 1999.

Brock, Dan. "Cloning Human Beings: An Assessment of the Ethical Issues Pro and Con." In *Cloning and the Future of the Human Embryo Research*, edited by Paul Lauritzen, 93-113. New York: Oxford University Press, 2001.

Brock, Dan. "Human Cloning and Our Sense of Self," *Science* 296 (2002): 314-316.

Brock, Dan. "The Non-Identity Problem and Genetic Harms – The Case of Wrongful Handicaps." *Bioethics* 9, nos. 3-4 (1995): 269-275.

Brock, Stephen L. "Is Uniqueness at the Root of Personal Dignity? John Crosby and Thomas Aquinas." *The Thomist* 69 (2005): 173-201.

Bruder, Carl E. G., Arkadiusz Piotrowski, Antoinet A. C. J. Gijsbers, Robin Andersson, Stephen Erickson, Teresita Diaz de Ståhl, Uwe Menzel, Johanna Sandgren, Desiree von Tell, Andrzej Poplawski, Michael Crowley, Chiquito Crasto, E. Christopher Partridge, Hemant Tiwari, David B. Allison, Jan Komorowski, Gert-Jan B. van Ommen, Dorret I. Boomsma, Nancy L. Pedersen, Johan T. den Dunnen, Karin Wirdefeldt, and Jan P. Dumanski. "Phenotypically Concordant and Discordant Monozygotic Twins Display Different DNA Copy-Number-Variation Profiles." *The American Journal of Human Genetics* 82, no. 3 (2008): 763-771.

Buber, Martin. *I and Thou*. New York: Charles Scribner's Sons, 1958.

Buchanan, Allen, Dan W. Brock, Norman Daniels, and Daniel Wikler. *From Chance to Choose: Genetics and Justice*. Cambridge: Cambridge University Press, 2001.

Burkhardt, Richard W. Jr. "Lamarck, Evolution, and the Inheritance of Acquired Characters." *Genetics* 194, no. 4 (2013): 793-805.

Burley, Justine, and John Harris. "Human Cloning and Child Welfare." *Journal of Medical Ethics* 25 (1999): 108-113.

Canellopoulou-Bottis, Maria. "Comment on a View Favouring Ignorance of Genetic Information: Confidentiality, Autonomy, Beneficence and the Right Not to Know." *European Journal of Health Law* 2 (2000): 185-191.

Cascais, A. F. "Bioethics: History, Scope, Object." *Global Bioethics* 10, nos. 1-4 (1997): 9-24.

Chadwick, Ruth. "The Philosophy of the Right to Know and the Right Not to Know." In *The Right to Know and the Right not to Know: Genetic Privacy and Responsibility* (Avebury Series in Philosophy), edited by Ruth Chadwick, Mairi Levitt, and Darren Shickle, 13-22. Aldershot: Ashgate, 1997.

Chapman, Audrey, and Jessica Wyndham. "A Human Right to Science." *Science* 340, no. 6138 (2013): 1291.

Chelouche, Tessa, and Geoffrey Brahmer. *Casebook on Bioethics and the Holocaust*. Haifa: UNESCO Chair in Bioethics, 2013.

Chousou, Dimitra, Daniela Theodoridou, George Boutlas, Anna Batistatou, Christos Yapijakis, and Maria Syrrou. "Eugenics between Darwin's Era and the Holocaust." *Conatus – Journal of Philosophy* 4, no. 2 (2019): 171-204.

Church, George, and Ed Regis. *Regenesis: How Synthetic Biology Will Reinvent Nature and Ourselves*. Basic Books, New York, 2012.

Cibelli, J. B., Ann A. Kiessling, Kerrianne Cunniff, Charlotte Richards, Robert P. Lanza, and Michael D. West. "Somatic Cell Nuclear Transfer in Humans: Pronuclear and Early Embryonic Development." *e-biomed: The Journal of Regenerative Medicine* 2 (2001): 25-31.

Cohen, Philip. "Cloning Humans May Be Impossible." In *The Ethics of Human Cloning*, edited by John Woodward, 54-56. Farmington Hills, MI: Thomson Gale, 2005.

Cohen, Shlomo. "The Ethics of De-Extinction." *Nanoethics* 8 (2014): 165-178.

Cohen-Almagor, Raphael. "Between Autonomy and State Regulation: J. S. Mill's Elastic Paternalism." *Philosophy* 87, no. 4 (2012): 557-582.

Costituzione della Repubblica Italiana. *Gazzetta Ufficiale* 298.

Council of Europe. *Additional Protocol to the Convention for the Protection of Human Rights and Dignity of the Human Being with regard to the Application of Biology and Medicine, on the Prohibition of Cloning Human Beings*. Paris: Council of Europe, 1998.

Council of Europe. *Explanatory Report to the Convention on Human Rights and Biomedicine*. Strasbourg: Council of Europe, 1997.

Cranston, Maurice. "Human Rights, Real and Supposed." In *Political Theory and the Rights of Man*, edited by David Raphael, 43-53. London: Macmillan, 1967.

Crosby, John F. III. "The Incommunicability of Human Persons." *The Thomist: A Speculative Quarterly Review* 57, no. 3 (1993): 403-442.

Crosby, John F. *The Selfhood of the Human Person*. Washington DC: The Catholic University of America Press, 1996.

Crosby, John F. III. "Why Persons Have Dignity." In *Life and Learning IX: Proceedings of the Ninth University Faculty for Life Conference*, edited by Joseph W. Koterski, 79-92. Washington DC: University Faculty for Life, 2000.

Davis, Dena. "Genetic Dilemmas and the Childs Right to an Open Future." *Hastings Center Report* 27, no. 2 (1997): 7-15.

Davison, Andrew. "Human Uniqueness: Standing Alone?" *The Expository Times* 127, no. 5 (2016): 217-224.

De George, Richard. "The Environment, Rights, and Future Generations." In *Responsibilities to Future Generations Environmental Ethics*, edited by Ernest Partridge, 157-166. New York: Prometheus, 1981.

Denaro, Pietro. "Moral Harm, Moral Responsibility, Ascriptivism." *Ratio Juris* 25, no. 2 (2012): 149-179.

Driesch, Hans. "Entwicklungsmechanisme Studien. I. Der Werth der beiden ersten Furchungszellen in der Echinodermentwicklung. Experimentelle Erzeugung von Theil und Doppelbildungen." *Zeitschrift für wissenschaftliche Zoologie* 53 (1891): 160-184.

Dunstan, Gordon Reginald. "The Moral Status of the Human Embryo: A Tradition Recalled." *Journal of Medical Ethics* 1 (1984): 38-44.

Düwell, M. "Human Dignity: Concepts, Discussions, Philosophical Perspectives." In *The Cambridge Handbook of Human Dignity*, edited by M. Düwell, J. Braarvig, R. Brownsword, and D. Mieth, 23-49. Cambridge: Cambridge University Press, 2014.

Dworkin, Ronald. "Rights as Trumps." In *Theories of Rights*, edited by J. Waldron, 153-167. Oxford: Oxford University Press, 1984.

Dworkin, Ronald. *Life's Dominion*. London: Harper Collins, 1993.

Dworkin, Ronald. *Taking Rights Seriously*. New York: Harvard University Press, 1978.

Eagan, Sheena M. "Normalizing Evil: The National Socialist Physicians Leagues." *Conatus – Journal of Philosophy* 4, no. 2 (2019): 233-243.

Egrie, Joan C. "The Cloning and Production of Recombinant Human Erythropoietin." *Pharmacotherapy* 10, no. 2 (1990): 3S-8S.

Eisenberg, Leon. "The Outcome as Cause: Predestination and Human Cloning." *The Journal of Medicine and Philosophy* 1, no. 4 (1976): 318-331.

Elliot, Robert. "The Rights of Future People." *Journal of Applied Philosophy* 6, no. 2 (1989): 159-169.

Emery, Gilles. "The Dignity of Being a Substance: Person, Subsistence, and Nature." *Nova et Vetera* 9, no. 4 (2011): 991-1001.

Engelhardt, Tristram Jr. *The Foundations of Bioethics*. Oxford: Oxford University Press, 1996.

Epictetus. *Discourses of Epictetus*. Translated by George Long. New York: D. Appleton and Co., 1904.

European Commission. *EU Charter of Fundamental Rights*, 2000.

Evans, M. J., C. Gurer, J. D. Loike, I. Wilmut, A. E. Schnieke, and E. A. Schon. "Mitochondrial DNA Genotypes in Nuclear Transfer-derived Cloned Sheep." *Nature Genetics* 23, no. 1 (1999): 90-93.

Evers, Kathinka. "The Identity of Clones." *Journal of Medicine and Philosophy* 24, no. 1 (1999): 67-76.

Feinberg, Joel. "The Child's Right to an Open Future." In *Who's Child? Children's Rights, Parental Authority and State Power*, edited by William Aiken, and Hugh LaFollete, 124-153. Totowa, NJ: Littlefield, Adams and Co., 1980.

Feinberg, Joel. "The Rights of Animals and Unborn Generations." In *Ethical Theory: An Anthology*, edited by Russ Shafer-Landau, 409-417. Oxford: Blackwell Publishing, 2007.

Feinberg, Joel. "Wrongful Life and the Counterfactual Element in Harming." *Social Philosophy and Policy* 4 (1987): 145-178.

Feinberg, Joel. *Freedom and Fulfillment: Philosophical Essays*. Princeton, NJ: Princeton University Press, 1994.

Feinberg, Joel. *Harm to Others*. Oxford: Oxford University Press, 1987.

Fiester, Autumn. "Ethical Issues in Animal Cloning." *Perspectives in Biology and Medicine* 48, no. 3 (2005): 328-343.

Finnis, John. "Some Fundamental Evils in Generating Human Embryos by Cloning." In *Ethics and Law in Biological Research*, edited by Cosimo Marco Mazzoni, 99-106. The Hague: Kluwer, 2002.

Fraga, Mario F., Esteban Ballestar, Maria F. Paz, Santiago Ropero, Fernando Setien, Maria L. Ballestar, Damia Heine-Suñer, Juan C. Cigudosa, Miguel Urioste, Javier Benitez, Manuel Boix-Chornet, Abel Sanchez-Aguilera, Charlotte Ling, Emma Carlsson, Pernille Poulsen, Allan Vaag, Zarko Stephan, Tim D. Spector, Yue-Zhong Wu, Christoph Plass, and Manel Esteller. "Epigenetic Differences Arise During the Lifetime of Monozygotic Twins." *Proceedings of the National Academy of Sciences* 102, no. 30 (2005): 10604-10609.

Freedman, Lynn, and Stephen Isaacs. "Human Rights and Reproductive Choice." *Studies in Family Planning* 24, no. 1 (1993): 18-30.

Gallin, Stacy, and Ira Bedzow, eds. *Bioethics and the Holocaust: A Comprehensive Study in How the Holocaust Continues to Shape the Ethics of Health, Medicine and Human Rights*. Cham: Springer, 2022.

Giles, J., and J. Knight. "Dolly's Death Leaves Researchers Woolly on Clone Ageing Issue." *Nature* 421 (2003): 776.

Gillon, Raanan. "Ethics Needs Principles – Four Can Encompass the Rest – and Respect for Autonomy Should Be 'First among Equals.'" *Journal of Medical Ethics* 29 (2003): 307-312.

Gillon, Raanan. "The Four Principles Revisited – A Reappraisal." In *Principles of Health Care Ethics*, edited by R. Gillon, 319-333. London: John Wiley, 1994.

Glod, William. "How not to Argue Against Paternalism." *Reason Papers* 30 (2008): 7-22.

Griffin, James. "First Steps in an Account of Human Rights." *European Journal of Philosophy* 9, no. 3 (2001): 306-327.

Griffin, Miriam. "Dignity in Roman and Stoic Thought." In *Dignity: A History*, edited by Remy Debes, 47-65. New York: Oxford University Press, 2017.

Grundgesetz für die Bundesrepublik Deutschland. *Bundesanzeiger* I, 968.

Guardini, Roman. *The World and the Person*. Translated by Stella Lange. Chicago: Henry Regnery, 1965.

Gurnham, David. "The Mysteries of Human Dignity and the Brave New World of Human Cloning." *Social and Legal Studies* 14, no. 2 (2005): 197-214.

Habermas, Jürgen. *The Future of Human Nature*. Cambridge: Polity Press, 2003.

Hadjantonakis, Anna-Katerina, and Virginia E Papaioannou. "Can Mammalian Cloning Combined with Embryonic Stem Cell Technologies Be Used to Treat Human Diseases?" *Genome Biology* 3, no. 8 (2002): 1023.1-1023.6.

Haldane, John Burdon Sanderson. "Biological Possibilities for the Human Species in the Next Ten Thousand Years." In *Man and His Future*, edited by Gordon Wolstenholme, 337-361. Boston: Little, Brown and Company, 1963.

Hall, Allan. "Hermann Goering's Great-Niece: I Had Myself Sterilized So I Would Not Pass on the Blood of a Monster." *The Daily Mail*, January 21, 2010.

Harman, Elizabeth. "Harming as Causing Harm." In *Harming Future Persons: Ethics, Genetics and the Nonidentity Problem*, edited by Melinda A. Roberts, and David T. Wasserman, 136-154. Dordrecht: Springer, 2009.

Harris, John, and Kirsty Keywood. "Ignorance, Information and Autonomy." *Theoretical Medicine and Bioethics* 22 (2001): 415-436.

Harris, John. "*Goodbye Dolly?* The Ethics of Human Cloning." *Journal of Medical Ethics* 23, no. 6 (1997): 353-360.

Harris, John. *On Cloning*. London: Routledge, 2004.

Harris, John. *Wonderwoman & Superman: The Ethics of Biotechnology*. Oxford: Oxford University Press, 1992.

Hart, Herbert Lionel Adolphus. *Essays on Bentham: Studies in Jurisprudence and Political Theory*. Oxford: Clarendon Press, 1982.

Hart, Herbert Lionel Adolphus. *Punishment and Responsibility: Essays in the Philosophy of Law*. Oxford: Clarendon, 1970.

Henley, Kenneth. "The Authority to Educate." In *Having Children: Philosophical and Legal Reflections on Parenthood*, edited by Onora O'Neill, and William Ruddick, 254-264. New York: Oxford University Press, 1979.

Hill, Thomas E. *The Blackwell Guide to Kant's Ethics*. Malden: John Wiley & Sons, 2009.

Hogan, Jennifer, A. Turner, K. Tucker, and L. Warwick. "Unintended Diagnosis of Von Hippel Lindau Syndrome Using Array Comparative Genomic Hybridization (CGH): Counseling Challenges Arising from Unexpected Information." *Journal of Genetic Counseling* 22 (2013): 22-26.

Holm, Sören. "A Life in the Shadow: One Reason Why We Should Not Clone Humans." *Cambridge Quarterly of Healthcare Ethics* 7 (1998): 160-162.

Hottois, Gilbert. "A Philosophical and Critical Analysis of the European Convention of Bioethics." *Journal of Medicine and Philosophy* 2 (2000): 133-146.

Huang, Ngan Tina. "The Ethics of Human Genetic Cloning." *MIT Undergraduate Research Journal* 4 (2001): 69-75.

Hutson, James H. "The Bill of Rights and the American Revolutionary Experience." In *A Culture of Rights*, edited by M. J. Lacey and Knud Haakonssen, 62-97. Cambridge: Cambridge University Press, 1991.

Huxtable, Richard. "Friends, Foes, Flatmates: On the Relationship between Law and Bioethics." In *Empirical Bioethics: Practical and Theoretical Perspectives*, edited by J. Ives, M. Dunn, and A. Cribb, 84-102. Cambridge: Cambridge University Press, 2017.

Institutes of Roman Law by Gaius. Translated by Edward Poste, revised by E. A. Whittuck. Oxford: Clarendon Press, 1904.

Jahr, Fritz. "Bio-Ethik. Eine Umschau über die ethischen Beziehungen des Menschen zu Tier und Pflanze." *Kosmos: Handweiser für Naturfreunde* 24, no. 1 (1927): 2-4.

Jennings, Herbert Spencer. "Heredity, Variation and Evolution in Protozoa II. Heredity and Variation of Size and Form in Paramecium, with Studies of Growth, Environmental Action and Selection." *Proceedings of the American Philosophical Society* 47, no. 190 (1908): 393-546.

Jonas, Hans. "Lasst uns einen Menschen klonieren: Von der Eugenik zu der Gentechnologie." In Hans Jonas, *Medizin und Ethik – Praxis des Prinzips der Verantwortung*. Frankfurt am Main: Suhrkamp, 1987.

Jonas, Hans. *Philosophical Essays: From Ancient Creed to Technological Man*. Translated by L. E. Long, edited by Carl Mitcham. Englewood Cliffs: Prentice-Hall, 1974.

Jonas, Hans. *The Imperative of Responsibility: In Search of an Ethics for the Technological Age*. Chicago: University of Chicago Press, 1984.

Jones, D. A. "The Human Embryo in the Christian Tradition: A Reconsideration." *Journal of Medical Ethics* 31 (2005): 710-714.

Jonsen, Albert R. *The Birth of Bioethics*. New York: Oxford University Press, 2003.

Kant, Immanuel. "What is Enlightenment?" In *Immanuel Kant, Perpetual Peace and Other Essays*, translated by Ted Humphrey, 41-48. Indianapolis: Hackett Publishing Company, 1983.

Kant, Immanuel. *Groundwork for the Metaphysics of Morals*, edited and translated by Allen W. Wood. New Haven and London: Yale University Press, 2002.

Kant, Immanuel. *The Metaphysics of Morals*. Translated by Mary Gregor. Cambridge: Cambridge University Press, 1991.

Kavka, Gregory. "The Paradox of Future Individuals." *Philosophy & Public Affairs* 11 (1982): 93-112.

Kemp, Peter, and Jacob Dahl Rendtorff. "The Barcelona Declaration." *Synthesis Philosophica* 46, no. 2 (2008): 239-251.

Kfoury, Charlotte. "Therapeutic Cloning: Promises and Issues." *McGill Journal of Medicine* 10, no. 2 (2007): 112-120.

Kuhse, Helga, and Peter Singer. *A Companion to Bioethics*. New York: John Willey and Sons, 2009.

Kuhse, Helga. "Should Cloning Be Banned for the Sake of the Child?" *Poiesis and Praxis* 1 (2001): 17-33.

Kumar, Rahul. "Who Can Be Wronged?" *Philosophy & Public Affairs* 31, no. 2 (2003): 99-118.

LaBar, Martin. "The Pros and Cons of Human Cloning." *Thought* 59 (1984): 319-333.

Ladenson, Robert F. "Mill's Conception of Individuality." *Social Theory and Practice* 4, no. 2 (1977): 167-182.

Laurie, Graeme. "Protecting and Promoting Privacy in an Uncertain World: Further Defences of Ignorance and the Right Not to Know." *European Journal of Health Law* 7 (2000): 185-191.

Lee, Kenneth. "Can Cloning Save Endangered Species?" *Current Biology* 11, no. 7 (2001): R245-R246.

Leibniz, Gottfried W. F. von. "Primary Truths." In *Philosophical Essays*. Translated by Roger Ariew, and Daniel Garber. Indianapolis: Hackett, 1989.

Leibniz, Gottfried W. F. von. *Discourse on Metaphysics and Other Essays*. Translated by Daniel Garber, and Roger Ariew. Indianapolis, and Cambridge: Hackett, 1991.

Levine, Mark A., Matthew K. Wynia, Meleah Himber, and William S. Silvers. "Pertinent Today: What Contemporary Lessons Should be Taught by Studying Physician Participation in the Holocaust?" *Conatus – Journal of Philosophy* 4, no. 2 (2019): 287-302.

Levy, Neil, and Miana Lotz. "Reproductive Cloning and a (Kind of) Genetic Fallacy." *Bioethics* 19, no. 3 (2005): 222-250.

Lo, Bernard, and Lindsay Parham. "Ethical Issues in Stem Cell Research." *Endocrine Reviews* 30, no. 3 (2009): 204-213.

Locke, John. *An Essay Concerning Human Understanding*, edited by Roger Woolhouse. London: Penguin, 1997.

Lolas, Fernando. "Bioethics and Animal Research. A Personal Perspective and a Note on the Contribution of Fritz Jahr." *Biological Research* 41 (2008): 119-123.

Lotz, Miana. "Feinberg, Mills and the Childs Right to an Open Future." *Journal of Social Philosophy* 37, no. 4 (2006): 537-551.

Lu, Yingfei, Yu Zhou, Rong Ju, and Jianquan Chen. "Human-animal Chimeras for Autologous Organ Transplantation: Technological Advances and Future Perspectives." *Annals of Translational Medicine* 7, no. 20 (2019): 576-584.

Mackenzie, John S. "Rights and Duties." *International Journal of Ethics* 6, no. 4 (1896): 425-441.

Macklin, Ruth. "Can Future Generations Correctly Be Said to Have Rights?" In *Responsibilities to Future Generations Environmental Ethics*, edited by Ernest Partridge, 151-157. New York: Prometheus Books, 1981.

Macklin, Ruth. "Splitting Embryos on the Slippery Slope: Ethics and Public Policy." *Kennedy Institute of Ethics Journal* 4, no. 3 (1994): 209-225.

Maienschein, Jane. *Whose View of Life? Embryos, Cloning, and Stem Cells*. New York: Harvard University Press, 2003).

Malby, Steven. "Human Dignity and Human Reproductive Cloning." *Health and Human Rights* 6, no. 1 (2002): 102-135.

Mameli, Matteo. "Reproductive Cloning, Genetic Engineering and the Autonomy of the Child: The Moral Agent and the Open Future." *Journal of Medical Ethics* 33 (2007): 87-93.

Manhart, Reinhold. "Medizin-Nobelpreis für ein Teufelswerk." *MMW – Fortschritte der Medizin* 152, no. 41 (2010): 6.

Mascetti, Victoria L., and Roger A. Pedersen. "Human-monkey Chimeras: Monkey See, Monkey Do." *Cell Stem Cell* 28 (2021): 787-789.

Maunu, Ari. "Indiscernibility of Identicals and Substitutivity in Leibniz." *History of Philosophy Quarterly* 19, no. 4 (2002): 367-380.

McCarthy, David. "Persons and Their Copies." *Journal of Medical Ethics* 25 (1999): 98-104.

McTaggart, John McTaggart Ellis. *The Nature of Existence*. Cambridge: Cambridge University Press, 1988.

Mill, John Stuart. *On Liberty: Utilitarianism and Other Essays*, edited by Mark Philip, and Frederick Rosen. Oxford: Oxford University Press, 2015.

Miller, Jessica Prata. "Introduction to Special Cluster on Feminist Health-Care Ethics Consultation." *APA Newsletters* 5, no. 2 (2006): 2-3.

Mills, Claudia. "The Child's Right to an Open Future?" *Journal of Social Philosophy* 34, no. 4 (2003): 499-509.

Montague, Phillip. "The Nature of Rights: Some Logical Considerations." *Noûs* 19, no. 3 (1985): 365-377.

Moore, G. E. *Principia Ethica*, edited by Thomas Baldwin. Cambridge: Cambridge University Press, 1993.

Morales, Nestor Micheli. "Psychological Aspects of Human Cloning and Genetic Manipulation: The Identity and Uniqueness of Human Beings." *Ethics, Bioscience and Life* 4, no. 3 (2009): 43-50.

Morsink, J. *The Universal Declaration of Human Rights: Origins, Drafting, and Intent*. Philadelphia: University of Pennsylvania Press, 1999.

Mulkay, M. "Frankenstein and the Debate over Embryo Research." *Science, Technology and Human Values* 21, no. 2 (1996): 157-176.

Munsie, M., C. O'Brien, and P. Mountford. "Transgenic Strategy for Demonstrating Nuclear Reprogramming in the Mouse." *Cloning Stem Cells* 4, no. 2 (2002): 121-130.

National Bioethics Advisory Commission. *Cloning Human Beings: Report and Recommendations of the National Bioethics Advisory Commission*. Rockville, Maryland, 1997.

Nelkin, Dorothy, and Suzan Lindee. *The DNA Mystique: The Gene as a Cultural Icon*. New York: W. H. Freeman and Company, 1995.

Newman, John Henry. "The Individuality of the Soul." *Parochial And Plain Sermons*. San Francisco: Ignatius Press, 1997.

Nozick, Robert. *Anarchy, State and Utopia*. Oxford: Blackwell, 1974.

Nussbaum, Martha. *Frontiers of Justice: Disability, Nationality, Species Membership*. Cambridge, MA: Harvard University Press, 2006.

O'Mathúna, Dónal P. "Bioethics and Biotechnology." *Cytotechnology* 53, nos. 1-3 (2007): 113-119.

Official Journal of the European Union, C 303/17 - 14.12.2007.

Offit, Paul A. *Vaccinated*. New York: Harper Collins, 2007.

Orentliche, David. "Beyond Cloning: Expanding Reproductive Options for Same-sex Couples." *Brooklyn Law Review* 66, no. 3 (2001): 651-683.

Ost, David E. "The 'Right' Not to Know." *The Journal of Medicine and Philosophy* 9 (1984): 301-312.

Palenčár, Marián. "Some Remarks on the Concept and Intellectual History of Human Dignity." *Human Affairs* 26 (2016): 462-477.

Parfit, Derek. *Reasons and Persons*. Oxford: Clarendon Press, 1987.

Pence, Gregory E. *Who's Afraid of Human Cloning?* New York: Rowman and Littlefield, 1998.

Peonidis, Filimon. "Making Sense of Dignity: A Starting Point." *Conatus – Journal of Philosophy* 5, no. 1 (2020): 85-100.

Perry, Michael J. "The Morality of Human Rights." *San Diego Law Review* 50, no. 4 (2013): 775-812.

Piechowiak, Marek. "Thomas Aquinas – Human Dignity and Conscience as a Basis for Restricting Legal Obligations." *Diametros* 47 (2016): 64-83.

Plachot, Michelle. "The Blastocyst." *Human Reproduction* 15, no. 4 (2000): 49-58.

Pogge, Thomas. "The International Significance of Human Rights." *Journal of Ethics* 4 (2000): 45-69.

Potter, Van Rensselaer. "Bioethics, the Science of Survival." *Perspectives in Biology and Medicine* 14, no. 1 (1970): 127-153.

Potter, Van Rensselaer. *Bioethics: Bridge to the Future*. Englewood Cliffs, NJ: Prentice Hall, 1971.

Prather, R. S., and N. L. First. "Cloning of Embryos." *Journal of Reproduction and Fertility Supplment* 40 (1990): 227-234.

Quiñones, Jose Luis Guerrero. "Physicians' Role in Helping to Die." *Conatus – Journal of Philosophy* 7, no. 1 (2022): 79-101.

Raikka, Juha. "Freedom and the Right (not) to Know." *Bioethics* 12, no. 1 (1998): 49-63.

Rawls, John. "The Law of Peoples." *Critical Inquiry* 20, no. 1 (1993): 36-68.

Rawls, John. *A Theory of Justice*. Oxford: Oxford University Press, 1972.

Rawls, John. *Lectures on the History of Moral Philosophy*, edited by Barbara Herman. Cambridge, MA: Harvard University Press, 2000.

Rawls, John. *The Law of Peoples*. Cambridge, MA: Harvard University Press, 1999.

Raz, Joseph. *The Morality of Freedom*. Oxford: Clarendon, 1986.

Regan, Tom. "Empty Cages: Animal Rights and Vivisection." In *Animal Ethics: Past and Present Perspectives*, edited by Evangelos D. Protopapadakis, 179-196. Berlin: Logos Verlag, 2012.

Reich, Warren Thomas. "The Word 'Bioethics': Its Birth and the Legacies of those Who Shaped It." *Kennedy Institute of Ethics Journal* 4, no. 4 (1994): 319-335.

Reiman, Jeffrey. "Being Fair to Future People: The Non-Identity Problem in the Original Position." *Philosophy & Public Affairs* 35, no. 1 (2007): 69-92.

Rhodes, Rosamond. "Genetic Links, Family Ties, and Social Bonds: Rights and Responsibilities in the Face of Genetic Knowledge." *Journal of Medicine and Philosophy* 23, no. 1 (1998): 10-30.

Riggs, Arthur. "Bacterial Production of Human Insulin." *Diabetes Care* 4, no. 1 (1981): 64-68.

Roberts, M. A. "The Non-identity Fallacy: Harm, Probability and Another Look at Parfit's Depletion Example." *Utilitas* 19, no. 3 (2007): 267-311.

Robertson, John A. "A Ban on Cloning and Cloning Research is Unjustified." *Testimony Presented to the National Bioethics Advisory Commission*, March 14, 1997.

Robertson, John A. "Involuntary Euthanasia of Defective Newborns: A Legal Analysis." *Stanford Law Review* 27, no. 2 (1975): 213-269.

Robertson, John A. "The Question of Human Cloning." *Hastings Center Report* 24, no. 2 (1194): 6-14.

Robertson, John A. *Children of Choice: Freedom and the New Reproductive Technologies*. Princeton, N.J.: Princeton University Press, 1994.

Rollin, Bernard E. "Keeping up with the Cloneses: Issues in Human Cloning." *The Journal of Ethics* 3, no. 1 (1999): 51-71.

Routley, Richard. "Is There a Need for a New, an Environmental Ethic?" *Proceedings of the XVth World Congress of Philosophy* 1 (1973): 205-210.

Roux, Wilhelm. "Über die künstliche Hervorbringung halber Embryonen durch Zerstörung einer der beiden ersten

Furchungszellen, sowie über die Nachtentwicklung (Postgeneration) der fehltenden Körperhälfte." *Virchows Archive für Pathologische Anatomie und Physiologie* 114 (1988): 419-521.

Sandel, Michael J. "The Ethical Implications of Human Cloning." *Perspectives in Biology and Medicine* 48, no. 2 (2005): 241-247.

Santosuosso, Amedeo. "Freedom of Research and Constitutional Law: Some Critical Points." In *An Anthology on Freedom of Scientific Research*, edited by Simona Giordano, John Coggon, and Marco Cappato, 73-82. London, and New York: Bloomsbury, 2014.

Sass, Hans-Martin. "Fritz Jahr's 1927 Concept of Bioethics." *Kennedy Institute of Ethics Journal* 17, no. 4 (2007): 279-295.

Savulescu, Julian, and Evangelos D. Protopapadakis. "Ethical Minefields and the Voice of Common Sense: A Discussion with Julian Savulescu." *Conatus – Journal of Philosophy* 4, no. 1 (2019): 125-133.

Schaefer-Rolffs, Jos. "Integrative Bioethics as a Chance An Ideal Example for Ethical Discussions?" *Synthesis Philosophica* 53, no. 1 (2012): 107-122.

Schopenhauer, Arthur. *The Basis of Morality*. London, Aylesbury: Hazell, Wattson and Viney, 1903.

Seneca. "Epistle LXXI." In *Ad Lucilum epistulae morales*. Edited and translated by Richard M. Gummere. Cambridge, MA: Harvard University Press.

Shalev, Carmel. "Human Cloning and Human Rights: A Commentary." *Health and Human Rights* 6, no. 1 (2002): 137-151.

Shapiro, Beth. "Pathways to De-extinction: How Close Can We Get to Resurrection of an Extinct Species?" *Functional Ecology* 31, no. 5 (2017): 996-1002.

Shaw, George Bernard. *Maxims for Revolutionists*. London: Constable, 2012.

Siep, Ludwig. "Ethical Problems of Stem Cell Research and Stem Cell Transplantation." In *Progress of Science and the Danger of Hubris*, edited by Constantinos Deltas, Eleni Kalokairinou, and Sabine Rogge, 91-99. Munster: Waxmann, 2006.

Silvestri, Erika. "Lebensunwertes Leben: Roots and Memory of Aktion T4." *Conatus – Journal of Philosophy* 4, no. 2 (2019): 65-82.

Simpson, James Young. "The Relation of Binary Fission to Variation." *Biometrika* 1, no. 4 (1902): 400-407.

Singer, Peter. "All Animals Are Equal." In *Animal Ethics: Past and Present Perspectives*, edited by Evangelos D. Protopapadakis, 163-178. Berlin: Logos Verlag, 2012.

Singer, Peter. *Practical Ethics*. Cambridge: Cambridge University Press, 1999.

Skre, Alf Butenschøn, and Asbjørn Eide. "The Human Right to Benefit from Advances in Science and Promotion of Openly Accessible Publications." *Nordic Journal of Human Rights* 31, no. 3 (2013): 427-453.

Smith, Lawrence C., Vilceu Bordignon, Marie Babkine, Gilles Fecteau, and Carol Keefer. "Benefits and Problems with Cloning Animals." *The Canadian Veterinary Journal* 41 (2000): 919-924.

Smolensky, Kirsten Rabe. "The Rights of the Dead." *Hofstra Law Review* 37 (2009): 763-803.

Sodeke, Stephen O., and Wylin D. Wilson. "Integrative Bioethics is a Bridge-Builder Worth Considering to Get Desired Results." *American Journal of Bioethics* 17, no. 9 (2017): 30-32.

Solter, Davor. "Viable Rat-Mouse Chimeras: Where Do We Go from Here?" *Cell* 142 (2010): 676-678.

Spemann, Hans. *Embryo Development and Induction*. New Haven: Yale University Press, 1938.

Spitz, Vivien. *Doctors from Hell: The Horrific Account of Nazi Experiments on Humans*. New York: Scientific Publications, 2005.

Statman, Daniel. "Who Needs Imperfect Duties?" *American Philosophical Quarterly* 33, no. 2 (1996): 211-224.

Steger, Florian. "Fritz Jahr's (1895-1953) European Concept of Bioethics and Its Application Potential." *Jahr* 6, no. 2 (2015): 215-222.

Steinbock, Bonnie. "Wrongful Life and Procreative Decisions." In *Harming Future Persons: Ethics, Genetics and the Nonidentity Problem*, edited by Melinda A. Roberts, and David T. Wasserman, 155-178. Dordrecht: Springer, 2009.

Stepien, Barbara K., Samir Vaid, Ronald Naumann, Anja Holtz, and Wieland B. Huttner. "Generation of Interspecies Mouse-rat Chimeric Embryos by Embryonic Stem (ES) Cell Microinjection." *Protocols* 2 (2021): 100494

Stocker, Michael. "Acts, Perfect Duties, and Imperfect Duties." *The Review of Metaphysics* 20, no. 3 (1967): 507-517.

Stolerman, Dominic. "The Moral Foundations of Human Rights Attitudes." *Political Psychology* 41, no. 3 (2020): 439-459.

Strong, Carson. "Cloning and Infertility." *Cambridge Quarterly of Healthcare Ethics* 7 (1998): 279-293.

Strong, Carson. "Reproductive Cloning Combined with Genetic Modification." *Journal of Medical Ethics* 31 (2005): 654-658.

Takala, Tuija. "The Many Wrongs of Human Reproductive Cloning." In *Bioethics and Social Reality*, edited by Matti Hayry, Tuija Takala, and Peter Herissone-Kelly, 53-66. Amsterdam, and New York: Rodopi, 2005.

Takala, Tuija. "The Right to Genetic Ignorance Confirmed." *Bioethics* 13, nos. 3-4 (1999): 288-293.

The European Parliament. "Resolution on Cloning." *Official Journal C 034 02/02/1998, p. 0164.*

Thomson, Judith Jarvis. *The Realm of Rights.* Cambridge, MA: Oxford University Press, 1990.

Tooley, Michael. "Moral Status of Cloning Humans." In *Human Cloning*, edited by James F. Humber, and Robert M. Almeder, 65-102. Totowa, N.J.: Humana Press, 2010.

UNESCO. "Universal Declaration on the Human Genome and Human Rights." In *Records of the General Conference. Volume 1: Resolutions*, 41-46. Paris: UNESCO, 1998.

Tsiakiri, Lydia. "Euthanasia: Promoter of Autonomy or Supporter of Biopower?" *Conatus – Journal of Philosophy* 7, no. 1 (2022): 123-133.

UNESCO. *Universal Declaration on Bioethics and Human Rights.* Paris: UNESCO, 2006.

United Nations. "Proclamation of Teheran." In *Final Act of the International Conference on Human Rights.* New York: United Nations, 1968.

United Nations. *Report of the United Nations World Population Conference.* New York: United Nations, 1975.

United Nations. *Report of the World Conference of the International Woman's Year.* New York: United Nations, 1976.

Ustava Republike Slovenije. *Uradni list Republike Slovenije*, no. 33/91-I.

Vignon, Xavier, Yvan Heyman, P. Chavatte-Palmer, and J. P. Renard. "Biotechnologies de la reproduction: le clonage des animaux d'élevage." *Inra Production Animales* 21, no. 1 (2008): 33-44.

Viljanen, Valtteri. "Kant on Moral Agency: Beyond the Incorporation Thesis." *Kant-Studien* 111, no. 3 (2020): 423-444.

Waldron, Jeremy. "On the Road: Good Samaritans and Compelling Duties." *Santa Clara Law Review* 40, no. 4 (2000): 1053-1103.

Ward, Robert, Saul Krugman, Joan P. Giles, A. Milton Jacobs, and Oscar Bodansky. "Infectious Hepatitis: Studies of Its Natural History and Prevention." *New England Journal of Medicine* 258, no. 9 (1958): 407-416.

Warnock, Mary. *Is There a Right to Have Children?* Oxford: Oxford University Press, 2002.

Weismann, August. *The Germ-Plasm: A Theory of Heredity*. Translated by W. Newton Parker, and Harriet Rönnfeldt. New York: Charles Scribner's Sons, 1898.

Wellman, Carl. "The Nature of International Human Rights." In *The Moral Dimensions of Human Rights*, edited by Carl Wellman, 71-84. Oxford: Oxford University Press, 2011.

Wells, David N. "Animal Cloning: Problems and Prospects." *Scientific and Technical Review of the Office International des Epizooties* 24, no. 1 (2005): 251-264.

Wilcox, Clinton. "The Human Embryo: Potential Person or Person with Great Potential?" *Christian Research Journal* 40, no. 3 (2017): 1-8.

Wilmut, Ian, A. E. Schnieke, J. McWhir, A. J. Kind, and K. H. S. Campbell. "Viable Offspring Derived from Fetal and Adult Mammalian Cells." *Nature* 385 (1997): 810-813.

Wilmut, Ian, Keith Campbell, and Cristopher Tudge. *The Second Creation: The Age of Biological Control by the Scientists Who Cloned Dolly*. London: Headline, 2000.

Wilson, Jane. "To Know or not to Know? Genetic Ignorance, Autonomy and Paternalism." *Bioethics* 19, nos. 5-6 (2005): 492-504.

Wojtyla, Karol. "The Personal Structure of Self-Determination." In Karol Wojtyla, *Person and Act and Related Essays.* Translated by Grzegorz Ignatik. Washington DC: Catholic University of America Press, 2021.

Wood, Allen W. "What is Kantian Ethics?" In Immanuel Kant, *Groundwork for the Metaphysics of Morals.* Edited and translated by Allen W. Wood, 157-181. New Haven and London: Yale University Press, 2002.

World Medical Association. "Declaration of Helsinki: Ethical Principles for Medical Research Involving Human Subjects." *Bulletin of the World Health Organization* 79, no. 4 (2001): 373-374.

Yanagimachi, Ryuzo. "Cloning: Experience from the Mouse and Other Animals." *Molecular and Cellular Endocrinology* 187 (2002): 241-248.

Zagzebski, Linda. "The Dignity of Persons and the Value of Uniqueness." *Proceedings and Addresses of the American Philosophical Association* 90 (2016): 59-74.

Zagzebski, Linda. "The Uniqueness of Persons." *Journal of Religious Ethics* 29, no. 3 (2001): 401-423.

Zuolo, Federico. "Dignity and Animals. Does it Make Sense to Apply the Concept of Dignity to all Sentient Beings?" *Ethical Theory and Moral Practice* 19 (2016): 1-13.